Improving Pain Care for Service Members

Administrator, Provider, and Patient Perspectives on
Treatment, Policies, and Opportunities for Change

KIMBERLY A. HEPNER, JESSICA L. SOUSA, CAROL P. ROTH,
SHREYA S. HUILGOL, CHESTER JEAN, LUCY B. SCHULSON,
PRIYA GANDHI, NIPHER MALIKA, CHARLES C. ENGEL

Prepared for the Under Secretary of Defense for Health Affairs
Approved for public release; distribution is unlimited

RAND NATIONAL DEFENSE RESEARCH INSTITUTE

For more information on this publication, visit **www.rand.org/t/RRA1193-2**.

About RAND

The RAND Corporation is a research organization that develops solutions to public policy challenges to help make communities throughout the world safer and more secure, healthier and more prosperous. RAND is nonprofit, nonpartisan, and committed to the public interest. To learn more about RAND, visit www.rand.org.

Research Integrity

Our mission to help improve policy and decisionmaking through research and analysis is enabled through our core values of quality and objectivity and our unwavering commitment to the highest level of integrity and ethical behavior. To help ensure our research and analysis are rigorous, objective, and nonpartisan, we subject our research publications to a robust and exacting quality-assurance process; avoid both the appearance and reality of financial and other conflicts of interest through staff training, project screening, and a policy of mandatory disclosure; and pursue transparency in our research engagements through our commitment to the open publication of our research findings and recommendations, disclosure of the source of funding of published research, and policies to ensure intellectual independence. For more information, visit www.rand.org/about/research-integrity.

RAND's publications do not necessarily reflect the opinions of its research clients and sponsors.

Published by the RAND Corporation, Santa Monica, Calif.
© 2023 RAND Corporation
RAND® is a registered trademark.

Library of Congress Control Number:
ISBN: 978-1-9774-1041-2

Cover: U.S. Air Force photo/Airman 1st Class Collin Schmidt.

About This Report

Acute and chronic pain are common among service members, with musculoskeletal pain and injuries being the leading cause of nondeployability among active-duty service members. Given the significant implications for individual health and force readiness, providing high-quality pain care to service members has long been a priority of the Military Health System (MHS). Prior RAND research (*Assessing the Quality of Outpatient Pain Care and Opioid Prescribing in the Military Health System*) used administrative data to assess the quality and safety of pain care and opioid prescribing in the MHS, generated a set of quality measures that the MHS could adopt going forward, and identified strengths and opportunities for improvement in care provided to service members with pain conditions. In this second phase of the study, interviews with MHS administrators, providers, and patients provide valuable detail and context for those findings, along with on-the-ground perspectives on MHS pain care policies and guidance in practice. This type of qualitative research can play an important role in clarifying drivers of variability in the quality of care provided to service members and aspects of pain care that are not easily captured in administrative data, including patient-provider communication, shared decisionmaking about treatment options, care coordination across providers, and barriers and facilitators to receiving needed care. The resulting findings highlight strengths and potential areas for improvement and innovation in pain care across the MHS.

The research reported here was completed in August 2022 and underwent security review with the sponsor and the Defense Office of Prepublication and Security Review before public release.

RAND National Security Research Division

This research was sponsored by the Office of the Assistant Secretary of Defense for Health Affairs and conducted within the Personnel, Readiness, and Health Program of the RAND National Security Research Division (NSRD), which operates the National Defense Research Institute (NDRI), a federally funded research and development center sponsored by the Office of the Secretary of Defense, the Joint Staff, the Unified Combatant Commands, the Navy, the Marine Corps, the defense agencies, and the defense intelligence enterprise.

For more information on the RAND Personnel, Readiness, and Health Program, see www.rand.org/nsrd/prh or contact the director (contact information is provided on the webpage).

Acknowledgments

We gratefully acknowledge the support of our project monitor CAPT Kenneth E. Richter of the Office of the Secretary of Defense for Health Affairs. We also appreciate the valuable insights we received from our reviewers, Marie Jo Larson and Stephanie Holliday. We addressed their constructive critiques as part of RAND's rigorous quality assurance process to improve the quality of this report. We thank Lauren Skrabala for contributions to sections of this report, Laurence Ma for assistance in preparing the report, Teague Ruder for conducting analyses to assess quality of pain care, and Bella González for assistance with data collection.

Summary

Delivering high-quality pain care has long been a priority of the Military Health System (MHS). Acute and chronic pain conditions are common among U.S. service members, with about half of active-duty service members having one or more pain diagnoses, most often musculoskeletal pain (Bader et al., 2018; Reif et al., 2018). Musculoskeletal pain conditions and injuries can be disabling and are the leading cause of nondeployability among active-duty service members and, therefore, have a negative impact on force readiness (Flynn et al., 2017; U.S. Army Public Health Center, 2020). Furthermore, treating service members' *chronic pain*—typically defined as pain lasting three or more months—can be complicated by the co-occurrence of other conditions, such as posttraumatic stress disorder, traumatic brain injury, and substance use disorders (Blakey et al., 2018; Lew et al., 2009).

This report presents findings and recommendations from the second of a two-phase study on pain care quality in the MHS. In the first phase, we collected and analyzed MHS administrative data to assess the quality and safety of outpatient noncancer pain care and opioid prescribing in the MHS, identifying areas of strength and opportunities for improvement (Hepner et al., 2022). The second phase of the study drew on qualitative data from interviews with military treatment facility (MTF) staff who oversee or provide pain care and service members who received pain care at MTFs. The objective was to gain a clearer picture of the real-world implications of MHS practices and policies for delivering pain care from the perspectives of MTF administrators, providers, and patients. Such qualitative data provide additional detail and context for the administrative data captured in the first phase of the study—shedding light on practice differences and effective models of care that can guide strategies to ensure that service members receive timely, high-quality pain care that supports their individual outcomes and the readiness of the force.

Study Methods

The findings and recommendations in this report draw on interviews with 68 MTF administrators and providers of pain care and 54 service members who were receiving care for chronic pain.[1] To capture a variety of perspectives and experiences, we recruited interview participants from seven MTFs that varied by size, service branch (three MTFs located at U.S. Army installations, two at U.S. Navy installations, and two at U.S. Air Force installations), and quality of pain care, according to 11 administrative data–based quality measures.

---

[1] All study methods were approved by RAND's Institutional Review Board and concurrence review provided by the Defense Health Agency Headquarters Human Research Protection Office.

Key Findings

Our interviews with staff and service member patients yielded several findings that can inform MHS efforts to implement the Phase 1 study recommendations and enhance its ongoing initiatives to improve pain care for service members.

- Nearly all providers reported assessing the severity of pain symptoms, but only approximately half said they used a structured method to assess pain severity and the impact of pain on patient functioning. Structured approaches that make use of existing MHS tools can help ensure that decisions about treatment adjustments are based on data collected in consistent ways over time.
- Nearly all providers endorsed a shared decisionmaking approach to developing a pain treatment plan. Most patients cited positive experiences with shared decisionmaking, noting that they were offered a choice of treatment options, felt that providers explained benefits and risks, or believed their providers listened to their preferences. However, most patients reported that communication between their providers was less than adequate, and nearly one-quarter felt they had been treated differently because of some aspect of their background.
- Consistent with the stepped-care model, most prescribers shared that they were reluctant to treat chronic pain with opioids and preferred nonopioid medications (e.g., oral nonsteroidal anti-inflammatory drugs) or nonpharmacologic treatment (NPT).
- Despite the availability of physical therapy and the high level of support for NPT among providers, more than three-quarters of staff reported that patients faced barriers to accessing NPT.
- Staff reported training and treatment access as the most important facilitators of high-quality pain care, whereas patients found effective treatment and patient-centered care most important.
- Staff and patients recommended prioritizing increases in treatment access and availability to improve pain care.

Recommendations

The following recommendations draw on both our qualitative interview findings and our analysis of MHS administrative data and pain care quality, presented in the Phase 1 study report. The recommendations presented here are in abbreviated form, and the study findings and rationale for the recommendations are provided in more detail in Chapter 9.

Recommendation 1. Increase Integration of Effective Nonpharmacologic Treatment

Recommendation 1a. Increase Access to Effective Nonpharmacologic Treatment

NPT is a recommended first-line treatment option for chronic pain and is central to the MHS's implementation of a stepped-care model of pain treatment. More than three-quarters of staff described the limited availability of NPT as the biggest barrier to integrating these treatments into pain care. It is critical that MTFs ensure that staffing and appointment availability are adequate to meet demand for these treatments. In our interviews, providers were more likely to mention integrating certain types of NPT, such as behavioral health care or psychotherapy, for pain compared with the proportion of patients who reported receiving these NPTs. These findings highlight the need to increase access to NPT, particularly to underutilized, recommended types of NPT. Innovative approaches may have the potential to increase access to NPT and could include on-demand access to physical therapy for chronic pain patients, more unit-embedded NPT providers, making telehealth appointments (e.g., for cognitive behavioral therapy for chronic pain) more widely available or expanding service members' access to NPT through private-sector providers, and designating a staff member at each MTF to serve as an expert in treatment options and to support NPT integration and coordination. The MHS should assess whether there is adequate availability of the types of providers necessary to ensure timely access to NPT.

Recommendation 1b. Monitor Access to Nonpharmacologic Treatment as Part of a Comprehensive Strategy to Improve the Quality of Pain Care

Ongoing monitoring of access and quality of care is essential to improving pain care in the MHS and can be used to ensure that care is delivered equitably across the patient population. Both phases of this study consistently found that service members received certain types of NPT (e.g., physical therapy) much more often than other types of NPT that were also recommended by the pain care research literature, such as acupuncture and psychotherapy associated with a pain diagnosis (Hepner et al., 2022). Using pharmacy data, the MHS monitors several metrics related to opioid prescribing at MTFs and by private-sector providers that contract with TRICARE (U.S. Department of Defense, 2021). Perhaps because of this ongoing monitoring, the MHS performs quite well across most metrics related to appropriate opioid prescribing. There is an opportunity to similarly expand these monitoring and improvement efforts to NPT integration. Phase 1 of this study generated several quality metrics related to monitoring NPT delivery (Hepner et al., 2022). There is an opportunity for the MHS to incorporate NPT into its ongoing efforts to standardize and track pain care. Doing so would help the MHS monitor access to specific types of NPT.

Recommendation 2. Identify Barriers to Broader Use of the Defense and Veterans Pain Rating Scale

The Defense and Veterans Pain Rating Scale (DVPRS) is the standard pain scale to be used by all providers (primary care and specialty) in MTFs to screen and assess for pain in adolescent and adult patients during each visit. Based on the intensity of pain, the DVPRS guides the assessment of pain's impact on the service member's functioning. The MHS has rolled out the DVPRS to providers, yet our findings suggest that continued support is needed to increase use of the DVPRS. Specifically, only half of providers reported using a structured method to assess the impact of pain on patient functioning and response to treatment. The reasons for the lack of use of the DVPRS to assess the impact of pain on functioning are unclear, and further work is needed to understand the specific barriers impeding broader implementation of the DVPRS. It is possible that providers could benefit from additional education on the use of the DVPRS and its value. In addition, the DVPRS should be feasible to use and easily accessible in the medical record. The current transition to GENESIS—the MHS's new electronic medical record—provides an opportunity to continue to promote the use of structured and longitudinal evaluations of outcomes of treatment and to provide other pain treatment decision support. The use of the DVPRS for standardized pain care assessment may also help to ensure that the pain care provided to service members is equitable.

Recommendation 3. Expand Provider Education on Effective Treatment Options and Appropriate Opioid Prescribing

Increasing provider training in targeted areas is a strategy that may help support the MHS in its ongoing quality improvement efforts. Staff endorsed the value of access to provider training and consultative support for pain care and recommended increased access to provider training and improved provider awareness of pain treatment options. To support this need, MHS should ensure that providers have protected time to attend training and that pain champions have time to support their providers.[2] MHS could also leverage existing programs, such as Project Extension for Community Healthcare Outcomes (ECHO), to achieve this aim.[3] Providers may benefit from MTF-specific guidance on available types of NPT, how patients can be referred, and whom to contact when faced with access challenges. Furthermore, providers may need additional training on appropriate opioid prescribing with an emphasis on how to prescribe for limited indications rather than solely on avoidance of prescribing. Most interviewed providers indicated some level of uncertainty and discomfort with prescribing opioids and, therefore, may benefit from additional guidance on when it is appropriate to prescribe opioids to treat service members with acute or chronic pain and

---

[2] *Pain champions* are primary care providers who receive specific MHS training on evidence-based pain management strategies.

[3] Project ECHO is a virtual training model in which primary care providers receive training to increase pain management competencies.

how to manage service members on long-term opioid therapy (LOT), including how to safely titrate patients off LOT, particularly given the risks of overdose and suicide risk with rapid titrations (U.S. Food & Drug Administration, 2019). Additionally, providers should be educated on when referrals to specialists should be made for complex opioid treatment cases based on a stepped-care model.

Recommendation 4. Explore the Feasibility and Impact of Allowing Extended Visit Length for Primary Care Appointments for Patients with Complex Pain Needs

Staff members identified inadequate appointment length as the most common overarching barrier to delivering evidence-based pain care. Staff explained that the standard appointment length of 15 to 20 minutes was generally inadequate, particularly for patients with complex pain care needs. Providers discussed needing more time during the visit to obtain patient buy-in, provide education, and discuss treatment options. Nearly one-quarter of staff members recommended that appointments for chronic pain patients be longer. Patients discussed the need for longer appointments to allow time to have their concerns addressed as part of the development of a treatment plan. Twenty-minute appointment times are often too short to manage preventive care and chronic medical conditions (Yarnall et al., 2003). Inadequate time may lead to further clinician burnout (Linzer et al., 2009) and potentially poorer quality of care (Linzer et al., 2015) and reduced patient satisfaction (Howie et al., 1991). The MHS should explore the potential impact and feasibility of defining an enterprisewide appointment standard that allows for a small number of complex patient appointments in primary care that would be longer than the standard appointment length of 20 minutes. Additionally, the MHS may consider expanding patient visit time by involving nurses or case managers as part of the visit for patients with chronic pain. These providers could support the primary clinician in patient pain assessment, education, and referrals.

Recommendation 5. Improve Patient Experience in Receiving Care for Chronic Pain, and Ensure Pain Care Is Equitable

Patients identified several positive aspects of their care for chronic pain received from the MHS, including shared decisionmaking, being offered a choice of treatments, learning about risks and benefits of treatment options, and feeling that their provider listened to their preferences. However, patients report less favorable perceptions of coordination of care between their providers, and nearly one-quarter felt they had been treated differently because of some aspect of their background (e.g., age or rank). These findings suggest that the MHS can continue to improve patient experience in receiving pain care and ensure that the care is delivered equitably. In addition, patients voiced a desire for more awareness of treatment options, including NPT and techniques for pain self-management. Interestingly, patients recommended increasing use of diagnostic imaging, such as magnetic resonance imaging, a perspective that is generally not consistent with recommendations in clinical practice guidelines. Increasing provider training and patient education materials would support providers in sharing evidence-based guidance on appropriate use of NPT and the role and timing of imaging in pain care. The MHS should also ensure that care is delivered equitably, particularly given persistent disparities in pain care in the United States (Hoffman et al., 2016; Institute of Medicine, 2001; Meghani, Byun, and Gallagher, 2012). Using stratified reporting, quality metrics can be used to examine variations in pain care (Fiscella, Burstin, and Nerenz, 2014; Health Research & Educational Trust, 2014; Jha and Zaslavsky, 2014; Meghani et al., 2012; Simon et al., 2015). Should care vary by patient characteristics, these variations should be investigated for potential causes and quality improvement strategies implemented to minimize variation. Providers and patients both referred to tensions between receiving appropriate treatment for pain and fulfilling military duties. Patient experience could be improved by directly addressing these tensions, such as through improving access to on-demand NPT or making it easier to schedule appointments around military training and work schedules. Some aspects of military culture may be associated with stigma toward service members who seek treatment for pain.

Conclusions

Our interviews with MTF staff and service members receiving treatment for chronic pain provided valuable context for the findings on pain care quality drawn from MHS administrative data in the first phase of this study. Administrative data capture patterns of care, offer insights into the extent to which service members receive evidence-based care, and are essential to measuring the quality of pain care in the MHS. Qualitative data provide a more nuanced picture of how the MHS organizes to provide pain care, how policies and guidance are implemented in practice, how patients experience pain care, and facilitators and barriers to high-quality pain care. The findings and recommendations in this report highlight areas for improvement and suggestions for innovation to ensure that the MHS continues providing timely, high-quality pain care that supports service members' outcomes and the readiness of the force.

Contents

About This Report... iii

Summary... v

Tables and Figures.. xiii

CHAPTER 1

Introduction... 1

    Providing Pain Care for Service Members... 1

    Phase 1 Assessment of Military Pain Care.. 4

    Contribution of Qualitative Interviews with Staff and Patients...................................... 10

    Organization of This Report... 11

CHAPTER 2

Methods... 13

    Interview Sample.. 13

    Interview Guides.. 15

    Data Collection.. 17

    Qualitative Data Analysis... 17

    Participant Characteristics.. 20

    Summary... 25

CHAPTER 3

Organizational Supports and Models of Care... 27

    Models of Pain Care.. 27

    Staff Perspectives on Approaches to Care and Models of Care...................................... 31

    Summary... 32

CHAPTER 4

Treatment Planning and Treatment Adjustment for Chronic Pain............................... 35

    Provider Perspectives on Initial Treatment Planning and Shared Decisionmaking......... 35

    Patient Experiences with Treatment Planning and Shared Decisionmaking................... 39

    Treatment Adjustment.. 45

    Assessment of Pain's Impact on Functioning... 47

    Patient Perceptions of Coordination of Care.. 49

    Patient Perceptions of Treatment Equity.. 51

    Summary... 53

CHAPTER 5

Pharmacologic Treatment for Chronic Pain... 55

    Prescriber Perspectives on Opioid Prescribing... 55

Processes to Support Providers in Prescribing Opioids 58
Challenges to Prescribing Opioids 61
Nonopioid Medication Used for Chronic Pain...................................... 63
Medications Avoided or Used Less Often for Chronic Pain 65
Medications Patients Received for Chronic Pain.................................. 65
Summary.. 67

CHAPTER 6
Nonpharmacologic Treatment for Chronic Pain................................... 69
Treatment Selection Considerations Specific to Nonpharmacologic Treatment 69
Nonpharmacologic Treatment Used or Avoided for Chronic Pain...................... 73
Staff-Reported Barriers to Nonpharmacologic Treatment 76
Processes to Support Providers in Integrating Nonpharmacological Treatment 81
Patient Perspectives of Nonpharmacologic Treatment............................. 82
Summary.. 84

CHAPTER 7
Facilitators and Barriers to High-Quality Pain Care 87
Facilitators and Strengths 87
Barriers.. 96
Summary.. 109

CHAPTER 8
Staff and Patient Recommendations 111
Interviewee Recommendations 111
Summary.. 124

CHAPTER 9
Findings and Recommendations.. 127
Strengths and Limitations 127
Key Findings... 128
Recommendations 131
Summary.. 138

APPENDIXES
A. Staff Interview Guide... 139
B. Patient Interview Guide 145
C. Selected Reviews of Effectiveness of Models of Care......................... 149

Abbreviations... 151
References 153

Figures and Tables

Figures

1.1   Percentage of Procedures or Service Members with Recommended Pain Care, by Quality Measure 6

5.1   Administrator-Reported Supports for Appropriate Opioid Prescribing 59

5.2   Nonopioid Medications That Prescribers Reported Using Most Often to Treat Chronic Pain 63

5.3   Medications That Patients Reported Taking to Treat Their Chronic Pain 66

6.1   Nonpharmacologic Treatment That Providers Reported Using Most Often to Treat Chronic Pain 74

6.2   Barriers to Incorporating Nonpharmacologic Treatment Most Frequently Cited by Staff 77

6.3   Nonpharmacologic Treatments That Patients Reported Receiving in the Previous Six Months 83

7.1   Facilitators Most Frequently Endorsed by Staff and Strengths Most Frequently Endorsed by Patients 88

7.2   Barriers to Pain Care Cited Most Frequently by Staff and Patients 97

8.1   Recommendations Endorsed by Staff and Patients 112

Tables

1.1   Quality Measures to Assess Pain Care 5

2.1   Criteria Informing the Selection of Military Treatment Facilities 14

2.2   Interview Domains 16

2.3   Characteristics of Staff Interviewees 21

2.4   Practice Characteristics of Staff Interviewees 22

2.5   Characteristics of Patient Interviewees 23

2.6   Patient Treatment Characteristics 25

3.1   Categories of the Most Common System Intervention Components 29

C.1   Selected Systematic Reviews of Effectiveness of Models to Deliver Multimodal Pain Care 150

CHAPTER 1

Introduction

Acute and chronic pain conditions are common among U.S. service members and are more common among military personnel than civilians (Sherry et al., 2021). Approximately half of active-duty service members have one or more pain diagnoses, with musculoskeletal pain being the most common (Bader et al., 2018; Reif et al., 2018). *Chronic pain*, typically defined as pain lasting three or more months, may be complicated by the co-occurrence of other conditions, such as posttraumatic stress disorder, traumatic brain injury, and substance use disorders (Blakey et al., 2018; Lew et al., 2009). Musculoskeletal pain conditions and injuries can be disabling and are the leading cause of nondeployability among active-duty service members and, therefore, have a negative impact on force readiness (Flynn et al., 2017; U.S. Army Public Health Center, 2020).

In the first phase of this study, RAND Corporation researchers assessed the quality and safety of outpatient noncancer pain care and opioid prescribing delivered to service members by the Military Health System (MHS) during fiscal years (FYs) 2018 and 2019 (Hepner et al., 2022). That work identified areas of strength in MHS pain care and areas for potential improvement. This report presents findings and recommendations from the second phase of the study, drawn from qualitative interviews with military treatment facility (MTF) staff and service members regarding pain care in the MHS. The objective was to provide a clearer picture of the real-world implications of MHS practices and policies for delivering pain care from both the provider and patient perspectives. The qualitative data provide a level of detail and context that cannot be captured in administrative data. Therefore, they can shed light on practice differences and effective models of care that can guide strategies for the provision of pain care going forward.

In this chapter, we provide an overview of efforts to improve pain care in the MHS and describe findings from the prior assessment of pain care delivered to service members. We conclude by describing how the qualitative interviews with MTF staff and patients extended our prior work and can enhance understanding of pain care delivery in the MHS.

Providing Pain Care for Service Members

Delivering high-quality pain care has been a priority of the MHS since the formation of the Pain Management Task Force in 2010. The task force was chaired by the Assistant Surgeon General for Force Protection and included appointed representatives from the U.S. Air Force, U.S. Navy, and Veterans Health Administration (Buckenmaier, 2010). The task force guides the implementation of policy and services to address service members' pain care needs, emphasizing multimodal and interdisciplinary strategies. These policies and resulting activities aim to ensure that adequate resources are available to facilitate patient-centered, evidence-based care for service members with pain; to ensure the provision of appropriate provider and patient education; and to support continued pain care research (U.S. Department of Defense and U.S. Department of Veterans Affairs, 2010).

Military Health System Policy Guidance

In 2018, the Defense Health Agency (DHA) issued the procedural instruction *Pain Management and Opioid Safety in the Military Health System (MHS)* to guide implementation of practices that support the MHS's goals regarding comprehensive pain care (Defense Health Agency Procedural Instruction 6025.04, 2018). This instruction included a guide to implementing the stepped-care model in patient-centered medical homes (PCMHs) and other primary care services to promote evidence-based pain management guided by clinical practice guidelines (CPGs). The guidance promoted the use of nonpharmacologic treatment (NPT) and minimized use of opioids. The instruction included prescribing guidance on opioids for treatment of pain related to outpatient procedures and management guidance for service members on higher opioid dosages or long-term opioid therapy (LOT) (Defense Health Agency Procedural Instruction 6025.04, 2018). The goal to provide effective pain care extended to strategically working with TRICARE contractors and facilitating the use of NPT and minimizing the use of opioids among service members who receive private-sector care.

The *Pain Management and Opioid Safety* instruction also aimed to facilitate the use of health information systems to guide and monitor pain care. It established the Defense and Veterans Pain Rating Scale (DVPRS) as the standard pain scale for use by all providers in the MHS's implementation of the stepped-care model (Defense Health Agency Procedural Instruction 6025.04, 2018). The DVPRS screens for pain and, based on intensity of pain, guides the assessment of its impact on the service member's functioning (U.S. Department of Defense and U.S. Department of Veterans Affairs, undated). The instruction also established the Pain Assessment Screening Tool and Outcomes Registry (PASTOR) as the designated screening tool and outcome registry for service members with chronic pain who receive tertiary-level care according to the stepped-care model and, potentially, for those who are escalated to secondary-level care (Defense Health Agency Procedural Instruction 6025.04, 2018). PASTOR includes the DVPRS and outcome measures of pain interference, physical functioning, anxiety, depression, and fatigue that allow for a more comprehensive assessment of factors related to chronic pain (Defense Health Agency, 2018).

In accordance with its goal to provide effective pain care, the MHS has committed to a policy that integrates behavioral health (BH) services into primary care settings to improve patient access to BH care (U.S. Department of Defense Instruction 6490.15, 2013; Defense

Health Agency Procedural Instruction 6025.27, 2019). Increased access to BH care is important for service members with chronic pain and comorbid BH conditions (Haibach et al., 2014). The MHS has also launched the Prescription Drug Monitoring Program to centralize data collection on controlled substances prescribed or dispensed to service members and has established procedures to ensure that prescribers and pharmacists can access and utilize the system when prescribing or dispensing controlled substances (Defense Health Agency Procedural Instruction 6010.02, 2021; Defense Health Agency Procedural Instruction 6025.04, 2018).

Pain Care Clinical Guidance

In addition to policies that support effective pain management, the U.S. Department of Veterans Affairs (VA) in collaboration with the U.S. Department of Defense (DoD) support best practices by maintaining CPGs for several common medical and BH conditions. The guidelines provide recommendations for care based on the strength of the evidence underpinning them (U.S. Department of Veterans Affairs and U.S. Department of Defense, undated). CPGs guide practitioners in patient evaluation and the development of evidence-based treatment plans. They also provide input on the development of quality measures to assess and monitor the degree to which care is concordant with recommendations. VA/DoD CPGs relevant to pain management include the following:

- *VA/DoD Clinical Practice Guideline for Opioid Therapy for Chronic Pain* (U.S. Department of Veterans Affairs and U.S. Department of Defense, 2022b; U.S. Department of Veterans Affairs and U.S. Department of Defense, 2017b). An update of the CPG issued in 2017 was released in 2022.
- *VA/DoD Clinical Practice Guideline for the Diagnosis and Treatment of Low Back Pain* (U.S. Department of Veterans Affairs and U.S. Department of Defense, 2022a; U.S. Department of Veterans Affairs and U.S. Department of Defense, 2017a). An update of the CPG issued in 2017 was released in 2022.
- *VA/DoD Clinical Practice Guideline for the Non-Surgical Management of Hip & Knee Osteoarthritis* (U.S. Department of Veterans Affairs and U.S. Department of Defense, 2020a; U.S. Department of Veterans Affairs and U.S. Department of Defense, 2014). An update of the CPG issued in 2014 was released in 2020.
- *VA/DoD Clinical Practice Guideline for the Primary Care Management of Headache* (U.S. Department of Veterans Affairs and U.S. Department of Defense, 2020b). At the time of this writing, this CPG was in the process of being updated.

DoD's work has taken place in the broader public policy context of the national public health crisis of opioid overprescribing and misuse. Therefore, in addition to VA/DoD, other agencies have issued guidance specific to pain care. Two of the CPGs that factored significantly into the quality measures for the Phase 1 study were being updated at the time of this writing and were published after this report was drafted in late 2022. The Centers for Disease

Control and Prevention's Clinical Practice "CDC Clinical Practice Guideline for Prescribing Opioids for Pain" was in draft form and available for public comment when we prepared this report, and has subsequently been published (Dowell, 2022). Similarly, the American Dental Association's guideline on the management of acute dental pain was being updated, with plans to publish in 2023 (American Dental Association, 2023). Its interim guideline emphasizes mandatory provider education on prescribing opioids, limiting the quantity of opioids dispensed, and the use of prescription drug monitoring programs to deter misuse and abuse (Garvin, 2018).

Phase 1 Assessment of Military Pain Care

To help readers understand the findings presented in this report, we begin with an overview of the RAND team's prior assessment of pain care delivered by the MHS to active-component service members (Hepner et al., 2022). We developed a set of 14 quality measures to assess outpatient care for acute and chronic pain, opioid prescribing, and medication treatment for opioid use disorder (OUD). This set of pain care quality measures was developed based on a review of existing measures, input from quality measurement experts, and suitability for use with MHS administrative health care data (Table 1.1). The measures were developed to be concordant with the recommendations of relevant VA/DoD CPGs, MHS procedural instructions, and key pain management guidance from organizations noted earlier. All guidance was current at the time of the study (i.e., 2018). The measures were used to assess quality of outpatient noncancer pain care provided by MTFs and private-sector care providers during FYs 2018 and 2019. The most common chronic pain conditions among service members in the Phase 1 study were low back pain (83.7 percent) and neck pain (24.6 percent) (Hepner et al., 2022).

Strengths and Areas for Improvement in Military Health System Pain Care

In this section, we provide an overview of the quality of pain care delivered by the MHS to service members from the Phase 1 study. Findings demonstrated both strengths and areas for potential improvement. Figure 1.1 summarizes the percentage of procedures or service members with recommended pain care.

Acute Low Back Pain

Three measures assessed care for a new episode of acute low back pain (Figure 1.1). Nearly 80 percent of active-component service members with acute low back pain received treatment consistent with stepped care; that is, these service members received an NPT or nonopioid medication in the three months after the initial visit and did not receive opioids or received opioids only after a trial of NPT or nonopioid medication. Treatment with

TABLE 1.1

Quality Measures to Assess Pain Care

Measure Topic	Quality Measure	Observed Care Phase 1
Acute Pain Related to Procedures		
Opioids and dental procedures	Dental procedures for opioid-naïve patients who initially received short-acting opioids and no more than a one-day supply or no opioids	FY 2019
Opioids and ambulatory procedures	Ambulatory procedures for opioid-naïve patients who initially received short-acting opioids and no more than a five-day supply or no opioids	FY 2019
Acute Low Back Pain		
Nonsteroidal anti-inflammatory drugs (NSAIDs)/NPT without opioids	Opioid-naïve patients with acute low back pain who received NSAIDs or any NPT within three months and no opioids	FY 2019
Stepped care	Opioid-naïve patients with acute low back pain who received nonopioids or any NPT within three months and no opioids or opioids only after nonopioids or NPT	FY 2019
No initiation of benzodiazepines	Opioid-naïve patients with acute low back pain not currently taking benzodiazepines who did not initiate benzodiazepines (≥7 days) within three months	FY 2019
Chronic Pain[a]		
NPT	Patients with chronic pain who received any NPT within 12 months	FYs 2018 and 2019
Nonopioid medication/ NPT	Patients with chronic pain who received any nonopioid medication or NPT within 12 months	FYs 2018 and 2019
Opioid Prescribing		
Opioids without concurrent benzodiazepines	Patients who received opioids and who did not receive concomitant benzodiazepines (≥7 consecutive days) during the 12-month observation period	FY 2019
Lower-risk average daily dosage	Patients who received opioids and whose average daily dosage was <90 MME[b] during the 12-month observation period	FY 2019
No advance to LOT	Opioid-naïve patients who received opioids and who did not advance to LOT during the 12-month observation period	FYs 2018 and 2019
Naloxone in LOT at higher-risk daily dosage	Patients on LOT dispensed a daily dosage of ≥50 MME and dispensed naloxone within three months	FY 2019
Follow-up visit in LOT	Patients on LOT with a follow-up evaluation and management visit at least every 90 days	FYs 2018 and 2019
Urine drug testing in LOT	Patients on LOT who received drug testing at least once during the 12-month observation period	FY 2019
Opioid Use Disorder		
Medication for OUD[c]	Patients with OUD who received medication treatment for OUD during the 12-month observation period	FY 2019

SOURCE: Adapted from Hepner et al., 2022.

[a] Chronic pain included low back pain, neck pain, osteoarthritis of the knee or hip, and fibromyalgia.
[b] MME = morphine milligram equivalent. This measure was also computed for average daily dosage < 50 MME.
[c] National Quality Forum–endorsed measure.

FIGURE 1.1

Percentage of Procedures or Service Members with Recommended Pain Care, by Quality Measure

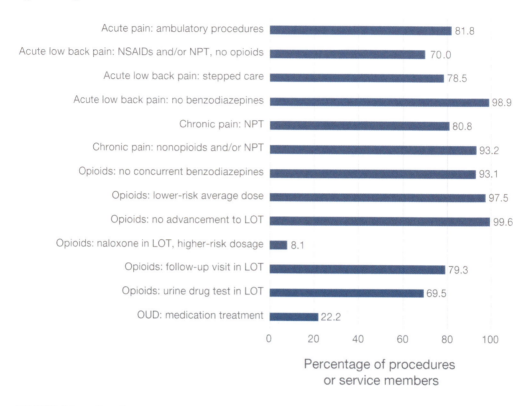

SOURCE: Adapted from Hepner et al., 2022.
NOTE: This figure does not include the quality measure addressing opioids after dental procedures. We had based the measure on a DHA policy regarding post-dental procedure prescribing that was under review at the time of this writing. Although performance on the measure was low (47 percent), our analyses of performance compared with recent consensus panel recommendations suggested that performance was higher. The measure score for Opioids: lower-risk dosage was also computed for average daily dosage less than 50 MME, which was 80.5 percent.

NSAIDs or NPT without opioids was high, and treatment with benzodiazepines was minimal (Hepner et al., 2022).

Chronic Pain

Nearly 100,000 service members experienced chronic pain in FY 2018 with low back pain being the most common condition. Of those with chronic pain, 37 percent had a BH condition, 29 percent had symptoms of a sleep disorder, and 36 percent were dispensed psychotropic medication. A subset of service members with chronic pain was identified as *high utilizers*, defined as the top quartile of health care utilization for this population. High utilizers had a median of 42 outpatient encounters in the observation year, including a median of six BH specialty visits and 21 non-BH specialty visits, and 70 percent had a BH condition.

These findings suggested a subpopulation of service members with chronic pain who are medically complex with high health care needs (Hepner et al., 2022).

Two measures assessed care for chronic pain (Figure 1.1). Among service members with chronic pain, 81 percent received at least one visit for NPT during the 12-month observation period. The most common NPT was physical or occupational therapy (75 percent), guided exercise (55 percent), and chiropractic care or manipulation (47 percent). Less frequently received NPT was acupuncture (7 percent), psychotherapy associated with a pain diagnosis (3 percent), and biofeedback or hypnotherapy (2 percent). It should be noted that other recommended forms of NPT are not recorded in administrative data and, therefore, would not have been available in the data analyzed for this study (Hepner et al., 2022).

Opioid Prescribing

Across most of the six measures assessing appropriate opioid prescribing, MHS prescribing adhered to practices that mitigated risk. For example, 93 percent of service members dispensed at least seven days of opioids had no concurrent use of benzodiazepines. Of service members prescribed an opioid, 98 percent had an average daily dosage below 90 MME and 81 percent had an average daily dosage below 50 MME. Less than 1 percent of opioid-naïve service members who were dispensed opioids progressed to LOT within 12 months. However, only 8 percent of service members on LOT who were dispensed opioids at a daily dosage of 50 MME or higher (and who were not dispensed naloxone in the prior two years) were dispensed naloxone within three months.

Medication Treatment for OUD

A single measure assessed the use of medication to treat OUD. Only 22 percent of service members diagnosed with OUD received any recommended medication treatment for OUD in that same year (Hepner et al., 2022).

Acute Pain Related to Procedures

For pain following minor outpatient procedures, DHA recommends an initial supply of short-acting opioids of five days or less. In FY 2019, 82 percent of the ambulatory procedures met this recommendation. When we compared MHS providers' prescribed initial total MME for the procedures studied to a recent consensus panel's recommendation for procedure-specific prescribing, performance across procedures was lower (49 percent), suggesting that the DHA recommended five-day supply may be generous for some procedures (Overton et al., 2018).[1] In the case of both ambulatory and dental procedures, guideline concordant care was higher

---

[1] At the time of the report, the DHA recommendation for initial opioid prescribing for post-dental procedure pain was no more than one day of short-acting opioids (Defense Health Agency Procedural Instruction 6025.04, 2018). This metric was met for 47 percent of dental procedures (Hepner et al., 2022). However, it should be noted that this recommendation was under review by the MHS at the time of the study. When compared with a recent consensus panel's recommendation on post-dental care prescribing, performance was 78 percent, suggesting that the DHA policy recommendation may be too stringent (Farooqi et al., 2020).

among direct care providers than private-sector care providers, and performance varied across procedures (Hepner et al., 2022).

Phase 1 Study Recommendations and Relevant Military Health System Activities

The findings from the first phase of this study supported six recommendations for optimizing pain care in the MHS. They are summarized here, along with some pain management activities reported by the MHS in its FY 2021 report on the implementation of its pain management policy (U.S. Department of Defense, 2021).

Use Quality Measures for Monitoring and Routine Reporting

Quality improvement efforts are facilitated by continually assessing whether patients received recommended care and providing feedback to providers. Therefore, we recommended that the MHS select a set of measures to use on an ongoing basis to establish benchmarks and track progress (Hepner et al., 2022). In its FY 2021 report, the MHS cited PASTOR and Military Orthopedics Tracking Injuries and Outcomes Network (MOTION) as two ways to longitudinally collect outcome data on service members with chronic pain and those with musculoskeletal conditions. PASTOR is prioritized for use in pain management clinics but may be used in primary or secondary care if desired by providers treating patients with chronic pain. MOTION is an enterprise system to link surgical and patient outcomes data for those with musculoskeletal injuries (U.S. Department of Defense, 2021). In addition, the MHS is monitoring high-risk opioid prescribing in both direct and private-sector care—specifically, average morphine equivalent daily dose (MEDD) equal or greater than 50 mg, co-prescription of opioids and benzodiazepines, beneficiaries on LOT, and high-risk patients on opioids who have been prescribed naloxone. MHS data have shown improving trends (i.e., decline in higher-risk opioid prescribing and increased naloxone dispensing) since 2017 (U.S. Department of Defense, 2021).

Increase Delivery of Recommended Nonpharmacologic Treatment for Pain

NPT is an essential part of the stepped-care model. We noted that although some forms of NPT were commonly received, others were less common. We recommended maximizing NPT availability and increasing beneficiary and provider awareness of NPT and non-opioid treatment benefits (Hepner et al., 2022). To this end, the MHS reported several pain management services for FY 2021. These include continued effort to provide clinical, education, and training support for pain management in primary care, including integrated BH consultants and primary pain care champions. Since 2019, providers in PCMHs have continued to implement a stepped-care model for pain and a clinical pathway to standardize the process of care and incorporate evidence-based pain management strategies. In 2020, the DHA issued new guidelines and regulations on the use of acupuncture to promote its use as a routine, complementary intervention (Defense Health Agency Procedural Instruction 6025.33, 2020). DoD and VA continue to partner with the National Institutes of Health's National Center for Complementary and Integrative Health on health research projects (U.S. Department of Defense, 2021).

Assess the Utilization Patterns of "High-Need" Service Members with Chronic Pain

We identified a subset of service members with complex cases of chronic pain who were high utilizers of health care and recommended assessing whether the needs of this population were being met (Hepner et al., 2022). As noted earlier, MHS's PASTOR and MOTION tools will enable longitudinal assessments and outcomes of patients as they move through primary, secondary, and tertiary levels of care, which can contribute to this assessment (U.S. Department of Defense, 2021). In addition, the DHA recently reiterated the required use of PASTOR in all MTF pain management clinics and indicated its intent to train one to three PASTOR subject-matter experts at each MTF pain clinic (Cordts and Defense Health Agency, 2022).[2]

Increase Naloxone Dispensing to Service Members with Higher-Risk Opioid Use

RAND analyses indicated that there were low rates of naloxone dispensing among those on LOT who had been dispensed opioids at a daily dosage of 50 MME or more (Hepner et al., 2022). The MHS has both the Prescription Drug Monitoring Program and the opioid registry. The latter includes decision support tools, such as calculated risk scores for opioid overdose; a patient look-up tool with specific recommendations for whether naloxone should be prescribed; and the Opioid Prescriber Trend Report that aggregates prescription data at the market, MTF, clinic, and provider levels (U.S. Department of Defense, 2021). A recent analysis of naloxone prescribing for MHS high-risk patients from January 2017 to February 2021 revealed that the probability of receiving a naloxone co-prescription was higher for patients whose opioid prescriber and pharmacy were both at MTFs versus when both were part of the private-sector care network (Pakieser et al., 2021).

Increase Medication Treatment for OUD

Because of military policies on drug use and substance use disorders, service members diagnosed with OUD are likely to be subsequently separated from the military (Army Regulation 600-85, 2020). Because of the low rate of medication treatment for OUD in the Phase 1 study population, we recommended offering medication treatment for OUD immediately following diagnosis and transition assistance programs to support separating service members to ensure continuity of care (Hepner et al., 2022). The MHS report on pain care management for FY 2021 did not specifically refer to medication treatment for OUD but did note that

---

[2] Jennifer L. Varney, Pain Management Clinical Support Services Chief, Defense Health Agency, personal communication with the authors, May 23, 2022.

the prevalence rate of OUD among active-duty service members fell from 0.15 per 1,000 in 2020 to 0.08 per 1,000 in 2021 (U.S. Department of Defense, 2021).

Update Opioid Prescribing Guidance for Procedures to Improve Specificity and Appropriateness

DHA policy on initial opioid prescribing for post-procedure pain is defined by a maximal number of days' supply (Defense Health Agency Procedural Instruction 6025.04, 2018). The Phase 1 analyses revealed high variability in performance for both dental and ambulatory procedures that was procedure specific and source specific (i.e., direct vs. private-sector care) with higher performance in direct care. Richard and colleagues (2021) found substantial variation in opioid prescribing for surgical dental procedures among dental clinics in the MHS from 2008 to 2017 (Richard et al., 2021). RAND recommended providing prescribing guidance that was more specific to quantity (total MME or quantity of specific tablets and dose) and to procedure (Hepner et al., 2022). Recent consensus panels have made recommendations for procedure-specific quantities of initial prescribed opioids for dental and select surgical procedures (Farooqi et al., 2020; Overton et al., 2018). Adopting procedure-specific recommendations for initial opioid prescribing was noted to be under DHA consideration for major procedures in 2018 (Defense Health Agency Procedural Instruction 6025.04, 2018). It is also supported by the Centers for Disease Control and Prevention's "Clinical Practice Guideline for Prescribing Opioids for Pain," which was available in draft form at the time of this writing and was subsequently published. This guideline notes the availability of procedure-specific opioid prescribing recommendations based on actual use and need data (Dowell, 2022).

This summary of Phase 1 study recommendations and related MHS activities is not exhaustive. It does not include all related MHS activities, such as training and education of health care personnel, patient education and information dissemination, service branch–specific activities, or ongoing research projects. It is noteworthy that in the intervening time since the prior RAND report, MHS activities and health care delivery were significantly affected by the coronavirus disease 2019 (COVID-19) pandemic. Most dramatic of these changes was the sudden increase in the proportion of outpatient visits delivered via telehealth rather than face to face (Hepner et al., 2023). It is unclear how these changes may have specifically affected utilization and delivery of pain care.

Contribution of Qualitative Interviews with Staff and Patients

While the first phase of this study used administrative data to assess the quality of pain care provided by the MHS in FYs 2018 and 2019 in both direct and private-sector care, this report focuses on findings from interviews with MTF administrative staff, providers of pain care, and service member patients receiving care for chronic pain. Because our interviews were limited to staff and patients at MTFs, we do not report themes on private-sector care. The interview participants came from MTFs that provided higher- and lower-quality pain care, according to administrative data–based quality measures. Qualitative data capture characteristics of care, such as details on the organizational strategies in care settings that support pain care provision, perceived barriers to care, and patient preferences, that cannot be derived from administrative data. An aim of this qualitative research was to better understand drivers of variability in the quality of care provided to service members, including organizational or system, provider, and patient factors. Additionally, qualitative interviews give an "on the ground" perspective on how and to what extent DoD policies and practices are implemented and insights into how and why these policies might be modified or diverged from. The interviews also helped illuminate reasons for patterns identified in the administrative data around the use of opioids, nonopioid medications, and NPT for chronic pain. Additionally, interviews with patients allowed us to characterize other aspects of pain care not easily captured in administrative data, including patient-provider communication and shared decisionmaking, care coordination, and equity. These data can be informative in identifying strengths and weakness in MHS pain care, drivers of variation in care, and potential areas for improvements and innovation in care.

Organization of This Report

This report describes the results of interviews with MTF staff (clinic administrators and providers) and active-duty service members regarding the provision and receipt of outpatient, noncancer pain care at MTFs. In Chapter 2, we outline methods used to select MTFs for study inclusion and to recruit interviewees. We also describe guides for interviewers, details of our data collection, qualitative analyses, and participant descriptive data. In Chapter 3, we provide a brief overview of effective models of pain care and staff perspectives on their general approaches to pain management. In Chapter 4, we present staff and patient input on planning and adjusting pain treatment and patient perspectives on shared decisionmaking, coordination of care across providers, and equity of care. In Chapters 5 and 6, we present staff and patient perspectives on pharmacologic and nonpharmacologic pain treatments, respectively. Chapter 7 focuses on staff and patient perspectives on supports and barriers to pain care, while Chapter 8 provides staff and patient recommendations for improving care. In the final chapter, Chapter 9, we summarize key findings and provide recommendations for the MHS for how to improve pain care delivery based on the findings from our work. In Appendixes A and B, we provide the staff and patient interview guides. Appendix C provides a summary of selected recent systematic reviews of multimodal models of pain care.

CHAPTER 2

Methods

In this chapter, we describe the methods used to conduct our study. We provide a description of our methods for selecting MTFs and recruiting both staff and patients at each MTF. We then describe our qualitative methods, including the interview guides used to structure data collection, along with the coding and analytic approach applied. Finally, we present characteristics of staff and patient respondents. All study methods were approved by RAND's Institutional Review Board, with concurrence from the DHA Headquarters Human Research Protection Office.

Interview Sample

In this section, we describe our approach for selecting MTFs, eligibility criteria, and recruiting staff and patients.

Military Treatment Facility Selection

We used a tiered stratified sampling approach that involved first selecting MTFs and then recruiting staff and patients from the selected MTFs. In April 2021, we selected seven MTFs from which to invite staff and patients to participate.[1] In selecting these MTFs, we aimed to maximize variation in quality of pain care. We selected a mix of MTFs with higher and lower performance based on a composite of selected pain care measures described earlier (Table 1.1). Specifically, we computed a mean of 11 measures assessing care for acute low back pain, chronic pain, and opioid prescribing for care delivered in FY 2018–2019 for each MTF. Measures assessing post-procedure prescribing and medication treatment for OUD were not included, as these aspects of care were not the focus on the interviews. In addition, we aimed to select MTFs representing a mix of service branches, sizes (defined as number of direct care visits in FY 2019), geographic locations, and whether the MTF had a pain clinic. We exam-

---

[1] We initially selected an eighth MTF, but ultimately the MTF was not included. The primary reason was related to the increased resources involved in conducting on-site data collection during the COVID-19 pandemic. Furthermore, the eighth MTF was an Army MTF, which was represented more than Air Force and Navy in terms of number of MTFs. We do not name the selected MTFs in this report, as we aimed to make recommendations for the MHS rather than specific MTFs.

ined these variables with the aim of increasing variability in pain care experiences rather than attempting to select a representative sample. Table 2.1 shows how we defined each characteristic, along with the number of MTFs in each category. By the time we conducted interviews in December 2021 to April 2022, the characteristics of these MTFs, such as quality of pain care, could have changed. We examined updated quality measure results assessing care provided in calendar years 2020 and 2021 and found that six of the seven MTFs remained in the same higher or lower performance tertile as with the earlier data; one MTF moved from the lower quality tertile to the medium tertile.

At the time of our interviews, the MHS was in the process of transitioning MTFs to using GENESIS, a new electronic health record (EHR). Two of the seven MTFs had incorporated GENESIS, and one was actively in the process of transitioning from the legacy EHR Armed Forces Health Longitudinal Technology Application (AHLTA) to GENESIS. The remaining four MTFs had not yet initiated this transition and were still using AHLTA.

Eligibility Criteria and Recruitment

At each MTF, we recruited staff and patients to participate in semistructured interviews. Eligibility criteria for staff were (1) being an active-component member of the U.S. military (Army, Navy, Air Force, or Marine Corps) or a DoD civilian and (2) being a provider or administrator involved in delivering or overseeing care for acute pain or chronic pain conditions at a selected MTF. Eligible providers included primary care practitioners, pain medicine specialists, integrated BH providers (e.g., psychologists, psychiatrists, or social work-

TABLE 2.1
Criteria Informing the Selection of Military Treatment Facilities

Characteristic	Description	Number of MTFs
Quality of pain care	Mean quality score derived by averaging quality measure scores assessing care for acute low back pain, chronic pain, and opioid prescribing for patients seen at the MTF in FY 2019, divided into three tertiles of MTFs defined as follows: • Higher: above 83% • Medium: 79%–83% • Lower: below 79%	Higher (3) Medium (0) Lower (4)
Service branch	Army, Navy, Air Force	Army (3) Navy (2) Air Force (2)
MTF size	Total number of direct care visits in FY 2019, divided into three tertiles defined as follows: • Large: more than 95,462 • Medium: 43,563–95,462 • Small: fewer than 43,563	Large (5) Medium (2) Small (0)
Pain clinic	MTFs identified by DoD as having a pain management clinic[a]	Pain clinic (5) No pain clinic (2)

[a] Identified by Medical Expense and Performance Reporting System 3rd level code BBL.

ers located in primary care settings), physical and occupational therapists, pharmacists, and other providers treating active-duty service members with acute or chronic pain in primary care or pain clinics. Examples of eligible administrators included chief medical officer, chief or deputy chief of primary care or pain medicine, pain committee chair, senior medical officer, and general practice manager. Eligibility criteria for patients were (1) being an active-component service member (Army, Navy, Air Force, or Marine Corps) and (2) reporting recent (i.e., in the past month) receipt of care for chronic pain (i.e., pain lasting at least three months) from the selected MTF. Eligible conditions included low back pain, neck pain, fibromyalgia, and other musculoskeletal pain (i.e., bone, muscle, or joint pain). Eligible clinics for patient recruitment were primary care, specialty pain care, and other treatment settings (e.g., sports medicine, occupational health, and physical or rehabilitative medicine).

We worked with points of contact at each MTF to identify eligible staff (up to eight providers and two administrators) and target clinics for patient recruitment. During planning calls with each MTF contact, we identified potential provider and administrator participants with a range of experience in direct care and oversight. At MTFs with designated pain clinics, we recruited staff and patients from both primary care and pain management clinics. We initially sought to conduct staff interviews during in-person site visits at each MTF. Because of the COVID-19 pandemic, we conducted some of our staff interviews remotely. Patient recruitment was conducted in person; we recruited a convenience sample of patients attending in-person appointments during the two or three days of on-site recruitment. MTF contacts were asked to post recruitment flyers in the waiting areas and examination rooms of selected clinics one week in advance of site visits. In identifying clinics for waiting room patient recruitment, we prioritized those with the greatest numbers of active-duty service member visits. Patient interviews were conducted in person or by phone.

To capture the range of experiences in primary care and pain management clinics in MTFs across service branches, we sought to interview up to ten staff (eight providers and two administrators) and ten patients at each MTF. Ultimately, we interviewed nine or ten staff and five to ten patients at each of the seven MTFs. Given the variation in pain care delivery across the MHS, we did not seek to reach thematic saturation (i.e., the point at which no new themes are identified). Instead, we sought to capture a range of staff and patient experiences to support an assessment of the barriers and facilitators to high-quality pain care across a variety of military treatment settings.

Interview Guides

We developed two separate semistructured interview guides for data collection with staff (providers and administrators) and patients (Table 2.2). Staff interview questions differed slightly between providers and administrators. Both guides were designed to capture respondent experiences and views relevant to key domains, including treatment approach; shared decisionmaking; treatment with NPT; medication treatment; treatment adjustment; and bar-

TABLE 2.2

Interview Domains

Interview Domain	Staff Interview Topics	Patient Interview Topics
Treatment approach	• Approach to pain treatment (providers) • Clinic or MTF approach to pain treatment (administrators) • Factors considered in developing a plan for treatment of chronic pain (providers)	• Coordination of care • Equity of care
Shared decisionmaking	Role of the patient in planning treatment for chronic pain (providers)	• Perceptions of discussions with provider(s) about different treatments • Treatment preferences and concerns
NPT	• Factors that influence use of NPT for chronic pain (providers) • NPT used most frequently or avoided (providers) • Degree to which providers at this MTF integrate NPT for chronic pain (administrators) • Biggest barrier to incorporating NPT • Processes to support providers in using NPT (administrators)	NPT for pain received in the past 6 months
Medication treatment	• Factors that influence use of opioids to treat chronic pain (providers) • Processes to support providers in appropriately prescribing opioids for chronic pain (administrators) • Medications commonly used to treat chronic pain (providers)	Medication treatments for pain received in the past 6 months
Treatment adjustment	• Factors considered in determining whether and how to adjust treatment (providers) • Assessment of how pain affects the patient's daily activities (providers)	• Assessment of pain impact on daily activities • Experience with changes to treatment in the past 6 months
Barriers	Barriers to delivering evidence-based treatment	Barriers to accessing quality care
Facilitators	Supports for delivering high-quality care	Facilitators and strengths of quality care
Recommendations	Recommendations to overcome barriers to care	Opportunities for improvement

riers, facilitators, and recommendations. Most questions included a series of follow-up questions (i.e., probes), most of which we attempted to ask consistently (see Appendixes A and B). Where appropriate, branching logic was used to tailor the guide to the respondent's experience or scope of practice (e.g., skipping medication questions for nonprescribers). Because our interviews were limited to staff and patients at MTFs, we did not include questions on private-sector care.

Data Collection

Interviews were conducted in person or remotely (i.e., by phone or secure web-based video conference) between December 2021 and April 2022. Interview duration ranged from 25 to 60 minutes. Both staff and patients provided verbal consent to participate. Interviewees were informed that participation was optional and that individual quotations would not be linked to the participant's name or MTF. Staff participated during on-duty hours and therefore did not receive an incentive. Patients who participated in an interview during off-duty hours could receive a $40 gift card.

To encourage participants to speak freely, interviews were not audio or video recorded. We conducted interviews in teams, with one team member taking electronic transcript–style notes. Team members conferred after each interview to review and finalize notes, ensuring de-identification and proper documentation of missing content (i.e., use of brackets to denote statements provided in explanation or to indicate gaps). Where possible, quotation marks were used in notetaking to indicate participant remarks that were believed to have been captured verbatim. Notes were stored on RAND file systems accessible only to research team members.

Qualitative Data Analysis

Interview note transcripts were cleaned and uploaded to Dedoose, a qualitative data analysis software explicitly aimed at facilitating rigorous qualitative research methods. A codebook was then created using the interview protocol and grounded theory method (a structured yet flexible research method that allows for discovery of emerging patterns in qualitative data) (Chun Tie, Birks, and Francis, 2019). Just as the interview guides differed for staff and patients, the codebook was developed to include different codes for these respondents. After multiple rounds of team discussions, the codebook was finalized and uploaded onto Dedoose for coding.

The coding team consisted of six individuals—three primary coders and three secondary coders. The secondary coders were used to ensure *intercoder reliability*, a measure that indicates the level of agreement between different coders. Intercoder reliability between two coders was 0.76 (across two transcripts), which was deemed acceptable based on the rule of thumb for acceptable reliability being 0.75 or higher (Norcini, 1999). Interviews were assigned to coders by interviewee type (staff or patient) to allow coders to develop in-depth knowledge of the content discussed by each type of stakeholder. At the start of the coding process, after one or two interviews were coded by both primary and secondary coders, the coding team met to resolve any discrepancies, ensure thorough understanding of the codebook, and address any questions. As coding progressed, weekly coding meetings were held to resolve any additional discrepancies.

After coding was completed, the coding team used thematic synthesis to analyze the data by exploring relationships and patterns between codes and respondent type (Thomas and

Harden, 2008). Codes were organized into descriptive themes and then further interpreted to yield analytical themes. In some cases, our descriptive themes may include overlapping concepts discussed in slightly different ways. In particular, we sometimes used different terminology for staff and patient respondents to reflect differences in the way different topics were described.

To facilitate our assessment of thematic content and differences across interviews, we assigned descriptor variables to each interview. Summary statistics on these variables are reported in the next section.

Descriptors assigned to all interviews are as follows:

- MTF name[2]
- interview modality
- service branch
- military status (military, DoD civilian)
- military rank.

Descriptors assigned to staff interviews are as follows:

- role (clinical, administrative, both)
- location of current clinical or administrative activities (primary care, pain management, physical occupational therapy/physical therapy/physical medicine/rehabilitative care, specialty pain care clinic, BH, other)
- provider type (primary care practitioner, pain medicine specialist, obstetric/gynecological physician, psychiatrist, psychologist, licensed clinical social worker, pharmacist, physical therapist, nurse [advanced practice or nurse practitioner], physician assistant, other)
- currently providing opioid medication treatment (yes or no)
- currently providing nonopioid medication treatment (yes or no)
- currently providing nonpharmacologic therapies (yes or no)
- currently providing management of long-term opioid use[3] (yes or no)
- currently providing medication treatment following procedures, such as surgical procedures (yes or no)
- number of years working as a military health provider
- frequency of care provided for patients with acute or chronic pain conditions, on average (multiple patients per day, multiple patients per week, multiple patients per month, one patient per month or less frequently).

---

[2]   Used to produce counts of results by number of MTFs only. MTF names and results for specific MTFs are not reported.

[3]   Defined as over 90 days of opioid medication therapy.

Descriptors assigned to patient interviews are as follows:

- race and ethnicity (American Indian or Alaska Native, Asian, Black or African American, Hispanic or Latino origin or descent, Native Hawaiian or Other Pacific Islander, white, none of these)
- military occupation
- gender
- age (18–24, 25–34, 35–44, 45–54, 55–64)
- patient diagnosed pain conditions (low back pain, neck pain, fibromyalgia, other musculoskeletal pain [bone, muscle, or joint pain])
- settings in which patient has received treatment for pain (primary care, occupational therapy/physical therapy/physical medicine/rehabilitative care, specialty pain care clinic, BH, other)
- duration of treatment for pain condition(s) (months)
- duration of treatment for pain condition(s) at this MTF (months).

We describe the prevalence of themes using consistent language to indicate the percentage of relevant interviewees that endorsed a concept. We use *a few* or *several* to describe themes endorsed by 10 percent or fewer respondents, using *a few* for only two or three respondents and *several* for four or five respondents. In addition, we use *one-quarter* for approximately 25 percent, *some* for 10 to 50 percent, *half* for approximately 50 percent, *most* for more than 50 percent, *three-quarters* for approximately 75 percent, and *nearly all* for 90 percent or more.

Exploration of the Positive Deviance Approach

We aimed to use a positive deviance approach to guide an assessment of differences in themes across staff and patients from the various MTFs but found our application of this method limited in several ways, decreasing its utility in our analyses. The goal of a positive deviance approach is to compare and contrast themes from positive and negative *deviant* sites (e.g., high- versus low-performing sites) in an effort to identify practices that are consistently present among positive deviants and absent among negative deviants (Rose and McCullough, 2017). This approach can help to identify what sites that are associated with top performance do differently from lower-performing sites, potentially identifying practices that should be promoted across sites (Bradley et al., 2009; Rose and McCullough, 2017). As described earlier, our seven sites included a mix of higher and lower performance on a set of pain care quality measures at the time of selection, but when we updated quality measure performance at the conclusion of data collection, one MTF had moved from the low to medium tertile. There are several reasons why results on the quality measures may not coincide with findings from our interviews. For example, our quality measures assess a variety of care delivered by MTF and private-sector providers, but our interviews were conducted only with staff and patients at MTFs. Furthermore, our interview sample likely included more staff and patients associated with pain clinics compared with patient care broadly characterized by our quality measures.

Thus, after reviewing potential findings and considering these significant limitations, we decided not to present findings from our positive deviance analyses.

Participant Characteristics

In this section, we describe characteristics of the staff and patients who participated in interviews.

Staff

Working with contacts at each MTF, we identified 76 staff for recruitment (ten to 13 from each MTF). We conducted interviews with 68 staff members (nine or ten from each MTF): 53 provider interviews and 15 administrator interviews. Of those who did not participate, two declined, three did not respond (i.e., no response after at least three attempts to schedule), and two were not eligible (i.e., they were not currently treating active-duty service members). Table 2.3 provides characteristics of participating staff.

Practice characteristics of staff interviewees are summarized in Table 2.4. Most staff worked in primary care (79 percent) or pain management (19 percent), and the majority were delivering or overseeing care for both acute and chronic pain at the time of our interviews. All provider interviewees were providing or referring patients to receive NPT. Most were prescribing nonopioid medication treatment (94 percent), medication for post-procedure pain (79 percent), or opioid medication treatment (77 percent). Nearly half were managing LOT (47 percent). Most reported treating multiple patients per day with acute or chronic pain (81 percent), whereas some reported treating multiple patients per week (18 percent). Among staff who participated in provider interviews, the average duration of clinical practice as a military health provider was 11 years.

Patients

We approached approximately 515 patients (35 to 120 at each MTF) through on-site waiting room recruitment to share information about the study and to inquire about patient interest and eligibility in participating in the study. We identified a convenience sample of 109 service members (11 to 22 from each MTF) who expressed interest in participating in an interview and whose initial responses during waiting room recruitment indicated study eligibility. Of those, we interviewed 54 patients (five to ten from each MTF). Among the individuals we recruited who did not participate ($n = 55$), 36 were lost to follow-up (i.e., did not respond after three attempts to schedule or reschedule), eight were not eligible (e.g., were not active-duty service members or did not have a chronic pain condition for which they had received treatment), eight declined (i.e., decided not to participate after providing their contact information in an initial expression of interest), and three were not scheduled because of having reached our maximum recruitment target of ten patients per MTF.

TABLE 2.3

Characteristics of Staff Interviewees

Staff Characteristics	Participants (*N* = 68)	
	%	*n*
Service branch		
Army	44.1	30
Navy	27.9	19
Air Force	27.9	19
Military status		
Active component	61.8	42
DoD government civilian	38.2	26
Rank		
O-3–O-4	44.1	30
O-5–O-6	17.6	12
N/A	38.2	26
Role		
Clinical only	41.2	28
Administrative only	4.4	3
Both clinical and administrative[a]	54.4	37
Provider type		
Primary care practitioner (MD, DO)	48.5	33
Pain medicine specialist	11.8	8
Psychologist	2.9	2
Nurse practitioner	11.8	8
Physician assistant	17.6	12
Other[b]	7.4	5

NOTE: DO = doctor of osteopathic medicine; MD = doctor of medicine.

[a] One respondent had both a clinical and administrative role but typically provided pain care to retirees and not to active-duty service members. We included this interview in the analysis because the interviewee provided information about their general approach to pain treatment and considerations for treating active-duty service members.

[b] Other provider types included a pharmacist, nurse case manager, clinical nurse supervisor, sports medicine physician, and orthopedic surgeon.

Table 2.5 provides characteristics of patient interviewees. As expected, based on the included MTFs, the largest cohort of patients were Army soldiers (41 percent), while the remainder were in the Air Force (28 percent), Marine Corps (17 percent), or Navy (15 percent). As required for eligibility, all patients were active-component service members. Most

TABLE 2.4

Practice Characteristics of Staff Interviewees

Characteristics	Participants	
Staff (N = 68)	%	n
Location of clinical or administrative activities[a]		
Primary care	79.4	54
Pain management	19.1	13
Physical medicine/rehabilitative care/occupational medicine/physical therapy	4.4	3
BH/substance use disorder specialty care	5.9	4
Pharmacy	1.5	1
Sports medicine	5.9	4
Other (e.g., acupuncture, orthopedics)	7.4	5
Delivering or overseeing care for[a]		
Acute pain conditions	100.0	68
Chronic pain conditions	98.5	67
Provider (N = 53)	%	n
Providing treatment for pain to service members at this MTF[a]		
NPT	100.0	53
Nonopioid medication	94.3	50
Medication for pain following procedures, such as surgical procedures	79.2	42
Opioid medication	77.4	41
Management of long-term opioid use[b]	47.2	25
Frequency of caring for patients with acute or chronic pain		
Multiple patients per day	81.1	43
Multiple patients per week	18.9	10
Combined	Mean	SD
Years working as a military health provider	11.4	8.0

NOTE: SD = standard deviation.

[a] Respondents could be included in more than one category.

[b] Long-term opioid use refers to over 90 days of opioid therapy.

were senior enlisted (E-5 through E-9; 67 percent). Based on the patient's reported military occupation, we categorized the occupation based on the level of physical demands, as this could be relevant to their pain care needs (Department of the Army Pamphlet 611-21, 2018). Most patients reported working in an area with moderate physical demands (e.g., Air Traffic

TABLE 2.5

Characteristics of Patient Interviewees

Patient Characteristics	Participants ($N = 54$)	
	%	n
Service branch		
Army	40.7	22
Navy	14.8	8
Air Force	27.8	15
Marines	16.7	9
Military status		
Active component	100.0	54
Rank		
E-1–E-4	20.3	11
E-5–E-9	66.7	36
O-1–O-3	3.7	2
O-4–O-8	5.6	3
W-1–W-4	3.7	2
Military occupation physical demand category[a]		
Work area with significant physical demands	18.5	10
Work area with high physical demands	7.4	4
Work area with moderate physical demands	64.8	35
Work area related to health care	9.3	5
Race and ethnicity[b]		
American Indian or Alaska Native	0	0
Asian	5.6	3
Black or African American	20.3	11
Hispanic or Latino origin or descent	25.9	14
Native Hawaiian or other Pacific Islander	1.9	1
White	50.0	27
None of these (specify)	7.4	4
Gender		
Male	74.0	40
Female	26.0	14

Table 2.5—Continued

Patient Characteristics	Participants (*N* = 54)	
	%	*n*
Age		
18–24 years old	9.3	5
25–34 years old	35.1	19
35–44 years old	40.7	22
45–54 years old	14.8	8
Pain conditions[b]		
Low back pain	88.9	48
Neck pain	44.4	24
Fibromyalgia	3.7	2
Other musculoskeletal pain		
Knee	46.3	25
Shoulder/elbow/arm	33.3	18
Ankle/foot	24.1	13
Hip	13.0	7
Hand/wrist/finger	11.1	6
Mid/upper back, rib	9.3	5
Joint pain, unspecified	7.4	4
Thigh/calf	3.7	2

[a] The level of physical demand required by the military occupational specialty (MOS) based on an assessment conducted by the Army. For more information, see (Department of the Army Pamphlet 611-21, 2018).

[b] Respondents could be included in more than one category.

Control Equipment Repairer and Human Resources Specialist; 65 percent). Half of patients identified as white (50 percent), one-quarter identified as Hispanic or Latino origin or descent (26 percent), and some identified as Black or African American (20 percent). Approximately three-quarters identified as male (74 percent) and one-quarter as female (26 percent). Most patients were aged 25 to 34 (35 percent) or 35 to 44 (41 percent). Consistent with prior findings from administrative data (Hepner et al., 2022), the most common pain condition reported by patients was low back pain, which was endorsed by 89 percent of patients.

Patient treatment characteristics are provided in Table 2.6. When asked about the types of settings in which they had received treatment for pain, nearly all patients mentioned primary care (91 percent) and occupational therapy/physical therapy/physical medicine/rehabilitative

TABLE 2.6

Patient Treatment Characteristics

Treatment Characteristics	Participants (*N* = 54)	
	%	*n*
In which types of settings have you received care for pain?[a]		
Primary care	90.7	49
Occupational therapy/physical therapy/physical medicine/rehabilitative care/human performance	94.4	51
Chiropractic/osteopathic	55.6	30
Specialty pain care clinic	55.6	30
BH	29.6	16
Complementary/alternative medicine—acupuncture, meditation, yoga, massage	14.8	8
Orthopedics	11.1	6
Surgery	7.4	4
Neurology/traumatic brain injury clinic	5.6	3
Neurosurgery/spine clinic	5.6	3
Ear/nose/throat	3.7	2
Podiatry	3.7	2
Rheumatology	3.7	2
Sports medicine	3.7	2
Deployed setting	1.9	1
Duration	**Mean**	**SD**
Months of receiving treatment for pain condition(s)	57.8	57.9
Months of receiving treatment for pain condition(s) at the selected MTF	20.3	28.9

[a] Respondents could be included in more than one category.

care (93 percent). The average duration of time receiving treatment for pain condition(s) at the MTF was 20.3 months.

Summary

In this chapter, we described the methodological approach we used for this study, including MTF selection, eligibility criteria, staff and patient recruitment procedures, data collection, and qualitative data analysis. We also presented participant descriptive data for staff and patients. We conducted interviews with up to ten staff and ten patients at seven MTFs with a mix of higher and lower performance based on a composite of selected pain care quality measures. This resulted in interviews with 68 staff (53 providers and 15 administrators) and 54 patients. Most staff were located in primary care or pain management clinics, and nearly all patients reported having received treatment for pain in primary care and occupational therapy/physical therapy/physical medicine/rehabilitative care settings. Approximately half of patients reported receipt of treatment in a specialty pain care clinic.

CHAPTER 3

Organizational Supports and Models of Care

To provide context for findings on approaches to pain care, we begin by providing a brief overview of recent systematic reviews of the effectiveness of models of pain care to better understand evidence of the effectiveness of various models. We also provide an overview of how the MHS stepped-care model and related MHS programs support pain care in the context of these models. Subsequently, we provide findings from our qualitative interviews with staff on their general approaches to treating pain.

Models of Pain Care

A model of care is a system-based means to deliver care that is evidence based, is concordant with CPGs, and results in improved patient outcomes (Briggs, Chan, and Slater, 2016; Peterson et al., 2017; Speerin et al., 2014). Models of care include interventions to support care delivery at multiple levels, including system (e.g., facility and funding), program (e.g., clinic), and specific component interventions (e.g., interventions of care, such as patient education and provider decision support) (Briggs, Chan, and Slater, 2016). In addition, the goal of implementing model components is to meet the needs of the patient population in the context of available operational resources: "the right care, delivered at the right time, by the right team, in the right place, with the right resources" (Briggs et al., 2012). The complexity of chronic pain calls for an interdisciplinary, multimodal approach to care (Briggs, Chan, and Slater, 2016; Defense Health Agency Procedural Instruction 6025.04, 2018; Haibach et al., 2014; Peterson et al., 2017; Institute of Medicine, 2011; U.S. Department of Defense and U.S. Department of Veterans Affairs, 2010). However, there is no standardized approach to describing and evaluating models of care in the literature (Guise et al., 2014). Various and evolving terms have been used to describe models or strategies for chronic pain management (e.g., multimodal, interdisciplinary, integrative, complementary, and self-management) (Guise et al., 2014; Kwon et al., 2021). In addition, model component interventions (e.g., decision support, education, and care management) vary in different settings in terms of the number of interventions and how they are implemented (e.g., distribution of CPGs versus incorporation of an EHR treatment template). These factors complicate the task of comparing models of pain care and determining the most effective interventions within those models.

Effective Models of Pain Care

We conducted a limited search of peer-reviewed literature to identify recent systematic reviews of effectiveness of models of pain care. We searched PubMed for systematic reviews focused on models of pain care for adult populations published between January 2012 and May 2022. The 106 articles identified were limited to 23 following title and abstract review. We selected five articles to discuss in this chapter (representing four systematic reviews— three with metaanalyses) (see Appendix C, Table C.1 for details on each review).[1] These four recent systematic reviews addressed the effectiveness of models of multimodal pain care but differed by populations studied, setting of care, and the model-component interventions evaluated. The studied population conditions included chronic musculoskeletal pain, neck pain and whiplash-related disorders, and fibromyalgia. The setting of care varied; some programs were situated in secondary and tertiary care, whereas others were in primary care or physical therapy (Elbers et al., 2022; Peterson et al., 2017; Peterson et al., 2018; Saracoglu, Akin, and Aydin Dincer, 2022; Sutton et al., 2016).

Models of Care and Outcomes from Systematic Reviews

All four reviews of the effectiveness of models of pain care assessed studies of multimodal care and measured patient outcomes. Peterson and colleagues (2017, 2018) reviewed system-based care for chronic musculoskeletal pain integrated in primary care. They included any intervention that sought to increase the uptake and organization of multimodal care (e.g., collaborative care, telecare, and stepped care). Given the heterogeneity of interventions associated with multimodal models of pain care, the authors grouped the most common interventions that targeted change in primary care processes for chronic pain management into four categories (Table 3.1). These categories were (1) provider decision support to enhance provider education and treatment planning, (2) additional care coordination resources, (3) improvement of patient education and activation, and (4) increased access to multimodal care (Peterson et al., 2017; Peterson et al., 2018). Of the nine models in these reviews, most included provider decision support and treatment planning. Five models that focused on decision support (mostly algorithm guided and/or stepped care) with proactive treatment monitoring demonstrated the best evidence for clinically relevant improvement in pain intensity and pain-related function over nine to 12 months but variable improvement in quality of life, depression, anxiety, and sleep (Peterson et al., 2018).

The remaining three reviews focused on variable modalities delivered in an interdisciplinary approach. Elbers and colleagues (2022) reviewed interdisciplinary multimodal pain treatment programs for chronic musculoskeletal pain that included a biopsychosocial model, treatment with active patient participation, at least three different health care professionals from various disciplines, and care provided via a single facility. Most programs included exercise, patient education, relaxation training, generic self-management skill training, and cog-

---

[1] Two articles are by the same authors (Peterson et al., 2017, and Peterson et al., 2018)—an evidence review and a related published article.

TABLE 3.1

Categories of the Most Common System Intervention Components

System Intervention Component	Example Interventions
Decision support to enhance provider education and treatment planning	• Facilitation of increased interaction between providers • Pain specialist peer support • Case management meetings • Risk triage • Stepped-care algorithms
Additional care coordination resources	• Health information technology mechanisms to collect and share information • Addition of a case manager into primary care • Addition of more frequent and regular patient monitoring
Improvement of patient education and activation	Increased breadth, intensity, frequency, and duration, of education and active patient engagement
Increased access to multimodal care	• Addition of previously unavailable services • Centralization of services

SOURCES: Peterson et al., 2017; Peterson et al., 2018.

nitive behavioral treatment. Program participation was associated with sustained improvements in physical and psychological well-being (Elbers et al., 2022).

Sutton and colleagues (2016) focused on neck pain and defined multimodal care as including at least two therapeutic modalities (e.g., acupuncture; patient education; exercise; manual therapy; and passive physical modalities, such as medication, assistive devices, psychological interventions, and soft-tissue therapies). The treatments associated with superior outcomes included exercise, manual therapy, and patient education, but evidence did not indicate that one multimodal package was superior to another (Sutton et al., 2016).

Saracoglu and colleagues (2022) reviewed the effectiveness of the addition of pain neuroscience education (a cognitive therapy designed to help patients understand and reconceptualize beliefs and attitudes about pain) to multimodal care for patients with fibromyalgia. The multimodal approach included basic patient education about fibromyalgia, exercise therapy, cognitive behavioral therapy, mindfulness training, and pharmacologic treatment. Metaanalyses showed that the addition of pain neuroscience education to multimodal care improved outcomes over multimodal care alone (Saracoglu, Akin, and Aydin Dincer, 2022).

Limitations of the Systematic Review

It should be noted that this brief review of models and the available systematic reviews has limitations. We aimed to highlight recent systematic reviews rather than conduct an exhaustive review. Systematic reviews of pain models were limited by the available studies and study quality. Additionally, these studies did not fully address certain factors that can affect effective delivery of pain management, including provider needs and constraints, patient modifiers, patient and provider preferences, shared decisionmaking, barriers to care, and facility factors (Peterson et al., 2018; Sokol, Pines, and Chew, 2021; Speerin et al., 2014; Suman et al., 2016). Finally, information about unintended consequences and burden of interventions was rarely reported (Peterson et al., 2018; Speerin et al., 2014). The reviews did not reveal a superior model of pain care but highlighted the variable complexity and quantity of interventions that may be associated with multimodal care. Peterson and colleagues organized common interventions into broader categories and highlighted the evidence for clinical improvement in programs associated with provider decision support and proactive treatment monitoring (Peterson et al., 2017; Peterson et al., 2018).

Military Health System Stepped-Care Model

In this section, we review several pain management activities reported by the MHS for FY 2021 (U.S. Department of Defense, 2021). Many of the MHS's efforts to support high-quality pain care align with the four system intervention components cited by Peterson and colleagues: (1) provider decision support to enhance provider education and treatment planning, (2) additional care coordination resources, (3) improvement of patient education and activation, and (4) increased access to multimodal care (Peterson et al., 2017; Peterson et al., 2018).

The MHS implemented the stepped-care model to promote evidence-based pain care guided by CPGs and promoting NPT, along with the appropriate use of opioids. The model provides a stepwise progression of care initiated in the primary care setting that guides initial treatment planning and subsequent treatment adjustment based on assessments of the patient's response to treatment. Patients whose pain is not responsive to primary or secondary treatment can be referred to specialty pain management clinics where available (Defense Health Agency Procedural Instruction 6025.04, 2018; Von Korff and Tiemens, 2000). The MHS reported further efforts to provide decision support in 2019 to 2021 through the continued implementation in PCMHs of a clinical pathway to standardize workflow processes and incorporate evidence-based pain management strategies with the support of specially trained primary care pain champions (U.S. Department of Defense, 2021). In addition, the MHS has initiated and standardized integration of BH services in PCMHs to facilitate collaboration between primary care and BH providers and increase patient access to BH care (Defense Health Agency Procedural Instruction 6025.27, 2019; U.S. Department of Defense Instruction 6490.15, 2013). Project Extension for Community Healthcare Outcomes (ECHO) uses telementoring to increase pain management competencies of remote primary care providers via secure audio-visual networks (U.S. Department of Defense, 2021). These examples illustrate some of the ways that the MHS targets provider decision support.

The MHS supports care coordination through its PCMH care managers. Several health care technology supports for sharing information include the Prescription Drug Monitoring Program and opioid registry, PASTOR, and MOTION (U.S. Department of Defense, 2021). The systemwide expansion of the GENESIS EHR provides a centralized medical record with patient portal and secure messaging with the health care team (Military Health System, 2022). Service-specific efforts aimed at patient education and activation include Army printed materials addressing pain awareness and Air Force patient education efforts to promote self-care strategies (U.S. Department of Defense, 2021). Examples of MHS efforts to increase access to care include the integration of BH care and pain care into primary care and increasing efforts to integrate pain telehealth for direct care visits (U.S. Department of Defense, 2021).

Although these and other efforts have been implemented in MTFs where care is system based and directly managed by the MHS, their application in private-sector care from TRICARE network providers is less clear. The 2018 DHA policy for pain management and opioid safety included a directive for the DHA Purchased Care office to work with contractors of private-sector providers to develop strategies to promote NPT and minimize opioid use in private-sector care settings (Defense Health Agency Procedural Instruction 6025.04, 2018). At the time of this writing, the MHS was monitoring high-risk opioid prescribing for TRICARE beneficiaries for direct and private-sector care through the Pain Management Clinical Support Service and shares opioid registry information with 46 states/territories (U.S. Department of Defense, 2021). Based on findings of the prior pain report, RAND recommended providing procedure-specific opioid prescribing guidance for all TRICARE prescribers (direct and private sector) (Hepner et al., 2022).

In summary, we conducted a targeted search for recent systematic reviews of the effectiveness of models of pain care. Reviews revealed no consistent terminology for describing the components of multimodal pain care, and care varied across settings in terms of the types, duration, and intensity of treatments included. In addition, other factors affecting pain care delivery, such as provider needs and constraints, patient characteristics and preferences, barriers to care, and burden of interventions, were not often examined. One review reported that pain care programs that included decision support with proactive treatment monitoring, a component of the stepped-care model, demonstrated the best evidence for clinically significant improvement. The same authors summarized the most common components of multimodal care as provider decision support, additional care coordination, patient education and activation, and increased access to multimodal care (Peterson et al., 2017; Peterson et al., 2018). Related to this summary, we cited recent MHS efforts in pain management that reflect activities concordant with these four components of care.

Staff Perspectives on Approaches to Care and Models of Care

As part of our interviews, we asked staff (administrators and providers) about their overarching approach to pain care, and whether it was structured or unstructured.[2] We also asked a subset of providers whether they typically used one treatment or multiple treatments at a time. Our goal was not to elicit an exhaustive list of components of care or the degree to

---

[2] All staff ($n = 68$) were asked about the approach to pain care at their MTF or clinic (for administrators, $n = 15$) or in their clinical practice (for providers, $n = 53$). Follow-up probes for nearly all staff ($n = 63$; both providers and administrators) queried whether that approach was structured or unstructured. An optional probe prompted most providers ($n = 47$) to describe whether they typically used one treatment or multiple treatments at a time.

which those components were used. Instead, we sought to obtain a general sense of each staff member's overall approach to pain care in preparation for a more detailed discussion of specific treatment considerations later in the interview, which are discussed in greater detail in subsequent chapters.

Approaches to Pain Care

Staff were asked to first describe their approach broadly to treating acute and chronic pain at their clinic or MTF or in their clinical practice (for administrators and providers, respectively). Staff commonly discussed several aspects of care (e.g., patient characteristics, past treatments, impact on functioning), which are presented in detail in subsequent chapters of this report. Many staff broadly referenced how CPGs or different models of care (e.g., stepped care) factored into their approach to treating pain. For example, staff mentioned a biopsychosocial pain model and a primary care pain management model. When describing the latter, one staff member commented, "We have essentially a pain management clinic and then we have pain management champions in each of our primary care clinics . . . [who] serve as the local subject-matter expert." We also asked staff whether the approach to pain care at their clinic or MTF (administrators) or in their clinical practice (providers) was structured or unstructured to understand whether a model of care guided their approach. The responses to this item were challenging to interpret. Many endorsed using a structured approach but did not mention a structured model. Respondents' endorsement of a structured approach may indicate use of a specific model of pain care; however, we did not specify criteria to define a structured approach, and therefore, the responses were based on respondents' interpretation of the question. A subset of staff explicitly referenced the stepped-care model. However, a sizable number endorsed using an unstructured approach, although a portion of these respondents mentioned the stepped-care model or another systematic approach to pain care. Regardless of whether they endorsed a structured or unstructured approach, staff referenced leveraging CPGs, tailoring approaches to their care settings and patient populations based on their clinical judgment, and integrating different providers and treatment types. Lastly, we asked a subset of providers whether they typically utilized one or multiple treatments at a time. Many stated that they employed more than one modality at a time; a few providers reported employing only one modality at a time. However, multiple providers stated that their use of treatments varied.

Summary

In this chapter, we summarized elements of effective models of care to treat chronic pain, described MHS policies and programs for pain management, and offered broad perspectives from staff on treating acute and chronic pain.

- **Models of pain care:** Although the systematic reviews that we highlighted differed in the reviewed programs' target populations, each included programs using multimodal models of care to treat chronic pain. The systematic review by Peterson and colleagues (2017 and 2018) focused on programs integrated in primary care, programs that have similarities to the MHS's stepped-care model. This review found that, among the multimodal pain programs reviewed, those with the best evidence of providing significant clinical improvement included provider decision support coupled with proactive, ongoing treatment monitoring. Additionally, they categorized the four most common system intervention components used in multimodal care to treat chronic pain: decision support (enhancing provider education and treatment planning), additional care coordination resources, patient education and activation, and increased access to multimodal care. We provided examples to illustrate how MHS policy supports these four intervention components of pain care. Although MHS efforts to guide opioid prescribing extend to both direct and purchased-care providers, other quality improvement efforts are mostly limited to MTF care.
- **Staff approaches to pain care:** Interviews with staff highlighted several factors that influenced their approach to treating acute and chronic pain. Staff endorsed employing both structured and unstructured approaches to pain care, although we did not inquire about the breadth and depth of implementation for either approach. Staff responses detailing unstructured approaches to pain care often aligned with those detailing structured approaches or references to the stepped-care model. Staff also discussed using one, multiple, or a varied number of treatment modalities, with differences driven by the patient context and provider clinical judgment.

CHAPTER 4

Treatment Planning and Treatment Adjustment for Chronic Pain

In this chapter, we describe findings on several themes related to treatment planning and adjustment for chronic pain drawn from provider and patient interviews. Chronic pain is persistent by nature, and patient needs vary over time. Given multiple treatment options, providers and patients need to agree on the plan for initial treatment and any needed subsequent adjustments to ongoing treatment. This chapter discusses both provider and patient perceptions of initial treatment planning and shared decisionmaking, treatment adjustment, and assessment of the pain's impact on patient functioning. We also describe patients' perceptions of coordination of care between their providers and issues of equity.

Provider Perspectives on Initial Treatment Planning and Shared Decisionmaking

In this section, we summarize themes related to provider perspectives on factors considered in developing an initial treatment plan, including the role of the patient in treatment planning.

Factors Considered by Providers in Developing a Treatment Plan

We asked providers ($n = 53$) about factors that they typically considered when developing a treatment plan for service members with chronic pain. Follow-up probes prompted providers to consider the role of patient factors (e.g., patient presentation or preferences), treatment factors (e.g., CPGs), and structural or organizational factors (e.g., clinic operations, policies, or programs). We also coded for provider-related factors (e.g., provider training or experience); however, this was not included as a specific follow-up probe.

Overall, the most common factors were the patient's clinical presentation (i.e., pain condition, severity, duration, impact on functioning, and presence of co-occurring BH conditions); service member responsibilities or career prospects; and treatment access or availability, particularly with respect to access limitations.

Patient-Related Factors

Most providers (n = 41) discussed the importance of assessing the type of pain condition, severity, duration, and impact on functioning or emphasized the importance of assessing for co-occurring BH conditions. As one provider stated, "[I consider the patient's] level of functioning, level of distress, comorbid issues—any other kind of comorbid diagnoses or mental health issues . . . a variety of factors." Additionally, half of providers (n = 27) mentioned the importance of evaluating the success of past treatments. As one provider stated, "[I ask patients], 'what have you tried, and what hasn't worked for you in the past?'"

Another common consideration mentioned by most providers (n = 30) was that of service member responsibilities and career prospects. Many of these providers commented on the importance of returning patients to a state of readiness for duty as quickly as possible. One provider explained,

> I would say one [of] the biggest things is, can I get them back on the ship, sub [submarine], or field? What can we do to get that done? That is what our mission is, because we're active-duty military. That is always my biggest concern.

Others emphasized the importance of understanding how aspects of the service member's military occupation influence their experience of chronic pain, such as for service members who were required to wear heavy gear or to make frequent airborne jumps or for those whose responsibilities precluded them from taking medications that could cause drowsiness (e.g., pilots, drivers, and those who carry a weapon). Others discussed the stage of the service member's military career (e.g., likelihood of deployment and proximity to retirement) as an important consideration.

About half of all providers mentioned the importance of patient preferences (n = 27), particularly with respect to desired treatments, and patient *motivation*, or willingness to engage in treatment. Explained one provider, "Some patients with chronic pain don't want to undergo invasive therapies to manage their pain; they prefer to manage it more conservatively. So, I take that into account." Additionally, half of providers (n = 27) mentioned other patient- or service member–related factors, such as age, deployment history, adherence to past treatment regimens, readiness for deployment, or patient knowledge about how to manage musculoskeletal injuries and acute exacerbations of chronic pain.

Organizational Factors

The second most common factor considered in developing a treatment plan was treatment access or availability, which was discussed by nearly three-quarters of providers (n = 38) across all MTFs. Most of these providers described barriers to the availability of treatment (n = 22), but others (n = 16) discussed the advantages of having certain treatments available to service members. Providers who reported access barriers referenced specific types of NPT that were limited or unavailable, whereas others mentioned difficulties accessing pain management specialists (particularly at MTFs with no pain clinic) or, less commonly, particular medications (e.g., nonformulary medications that require prior authorization, such as brand name Lyrica). As one provider at an MTF with no pain clinic shared,

> I guess availability of resources would impact treatment. How soon [can] a patient get in with somebody? Or, like, we don't have a chiropractor here currently. So that would play a role. And we don't have pain management specialists here, so we would have to refer them out [to see community providers].

Providers who mentioned the advantages of the availability of particular treatments seemed to indicate a greater awareness of how to access pain specialists or specialized treatments, although many still acknowledged that resources were finite. As one provider located in primary care at an MTF with a specialty pain clinic explained,

> If you're active duty, it's really lovely, because we have the pain management clinic here that has their comprehensive plan. So . . . you've got the interventionist who can do injections, you've got the psychologist, chiropractor, pain specialist doctors up here, they have a nutritionist, a yoga person, it's all right there, so if you're active duty, they probably don't even realize how awesome that is, but they have this incredibly comprehensive program offered to them.

Other providers who described treatment access or availability as an advantageous factor in treatment planning discussed having embedded BH providers available to support service members with chronic pain.

Some providers ($n = 6$) mentioned MTF policies or specific programs, such as a structured intake process for chronic pain or a telehealth service for pain medicine. Some ($n = 7$) also discussed care coordination (e.g., discussing treatment during clinic team meetings or conferring with treating providers in other clinics), and some ($n = 8$) mentioned the availability of consultation with a pain clinic, pharmacy, or other specialists. A small number of respondents mentioned additional considerations, such as appointment wait times ($n = 5$), military Medical Evaluation Board policy ($n = 4$), or inadequate staffing (i.e., undermanning; attrition of specific staff, such as physical therapists and psychologists) ($n = 2$).

Treatment-Related Factors

Some providers ($n = 21$) mentioned CPGs, citing them as helpful in guiding treatment planning. Specifically, providers referenced DoD guidelines for chronic pain management and for opioid prescribing. One provider explained,

> We look at the guidelines when it comes to, for example, occasionally prescribing opioids—mostly for the nonactive duty population—looking at the VA/DoD chronic opioid guidelines or the VA/DoD clinical guidelines for the treatment of low back pain. Things like that.

Additionally, one-quarter of providers ($n = 13$) discussed their perceptions of treatment effectiveness as being a consideration in treatment planning, referencing a preference for evidence-based therapies or an avoidance of treatments perceived as ineffective. One provider remarked, "opioids are proven to be noneffective, so I don't use them." Some providers ($n = 7$) mentioned treatment safety or side effects as an important factor in developing a treatment plan, particularly with respect to medications (e.g., "with patients that may use a lot of NSAIDs and have gastric problems, we try to stay away from excessive NSAID use for them"). Others ($n = 9$) discussed other treatment-related factors, such as measurement-based care or the use of a holistic treatment approach.

Provider-Related Factors

Provider-related factors considered in treatment selection included provider experience or background ($n = 10$), beliefs and preferences ($n = 6$), clinical judgment or discretion ($n = 5$), and provider post-professional training ($n = 4$).

Provider Perspectives of the Role of the Patient in Treatment Planning

We asked all providers ($n = 53$) whether the patient played a role in the treatment planning process for service members with chronic pain. As expected, most providers ($n = 48$) across all MTFs said that the patient played a role in the treatment planning process. However, several providers ($n = 4$) indicated that this varies by patient and by treatment. For example, one provider emphasized the importance of good communication and securing patient buy-in for ensuring compliance with treatment but explained, "[NPT] is part of the program. If there is a patient that resists—if there is somebody that just wants pills, I just don't entertain that. . . . That's my approach to narcotics." Another provider indicated that treatment for chronic pain tends to be structured and that this limits the extent to which patients might be involved in treatment planning. Only one provider stated that the patient does not generally play a role in the treatment planning process, explaining that their patients tend to come to the visit wanting to hear what the physician thinks is best for their treatment.

Among the providers who indicated that the patient plays a role in treatment planning ($n = 48$), responses with respect to how this occurred varied. Common themes included building patient buy-in and motivation for treatment ($n = 27$), providing patients with treatment options ($n = 25$), determining patient goals and priorities for treatment ($n = 25$), and educating patients ($n = 23$). One provider endorsed several of these themes, stating, "I always seek patients' input and offer multiple options. Because it really just drives their care a bit better and they're more compliant and more invested [in treatment]." In describing the importance of patient education for securing buy-in and motivation, one provider explained,

> If I say I'm going to send you for physical therapy and I hear a response, 'I really can't go, I have too much work to do,' [then] I need to educate them [the patient] that, 'this is going to help you, this is going to reduce your duration of symptoms.' Participation and educa-

tion are very important. If a service member is not receptive or not convinced that it is beneficial, they may not go. So, their participation and willingness are very important for their treatment.

Providers also mentioned offering several treatment options for chronic pain and their belief that this helped increase patient engagement or treatment adherence. One clinician explained, "I give [patients] options of what we can do. I tell my patients, 'We can be as aggressive or minimal as you want.'" Another stated, "I always seek patients' input and offer multiple options. Because it really just drives their care a bit better, and they're more compliant and more invested [in treatment]." Others discussed the importance of determining patients' willingness or comfort with engaging in a recommended treatment before deciding on a plan of action. As a part of this process, providers mentioned setting reasonable expectations or ensuring patient understanding of the prognosis and anticipated treatment course. Another provider described the importance of understanding the patient's treatment goals, explaining,

> For service members specifically, I think, when I treat any patient, you need to ask them their goals of care. . . . If you're giving active-duty soldiers opiates or Marinol [cannabinoid], these are things they cannot continue to take and still function in the military, so making sure to avoid those [medications]—otherwise, it will nullify their security clearance or impact their ability to do their job.

Additionally, some providers ($n = 19$) emphasized the importance of patient autonomy or patient choice, and some ($n = 11$) discussed the importance of the strength of the clinician-patient relationship (i.e., therapeutic alliance).

In conclusion, providers stated that the patient plays a role in the treatment planning process. The most common themes included the importance of building buy-in and motivation for patient engagement, determining the goals and treatment interests of the patient, and providing multiple treatment options.

Patient Experiences with Treatment Planning and Shared Decisionmaking

We asked patients with chronic pain ($n = 54$) about whether they recalled talking with any provider about different treatments for their pain and what they recalled about these discussions. In follow-up probes, patients were asked about their being offered a choice of treatments, receiving explanations about the benefits and risks of a treatment, and receiving recommendations from a provider regarding appropriate treatment, as well as their general experiences with providers listening to their treatment preferences. Most patients ($n = 34$) responded that they felt that they had discussed treatment options with their providers. Of those who were queried about whether their providers offered a choice of treatment ($n = 47$), slightly more than half (*n* = 25) felt that they were offered a choice of treatments. Patients who felt they had discussed treatment options with their providers reported that, oftentimes, their primary care manager (PCM) would give them an overview of the treatment options, including referrals to specialty care. A patient explained,

> [T]he doctor . . . was able to kind of talk to me about all of those [possible treatments]; she just asked me what I think the best course of action [would be] and she also gave me her opinion on what she thought would work.

One patient described the options as "escalatory," with providers offering less invasive treatments early on. Patients shared that their provider often recommended physical therapy as an initial referral, followed by other NPT. Other patients felt that they were offered more treatment choices in certain settings. A patient stated, "Specialty [pain] care was much better [than primary care in offering a choice of treatments]. They actually gave me options and were more than willing to work with me on what options to take and what routes to take to try to get a remedy." Many also patients described long wait times and slow referral processes to get appointments for treatment and diagnostic imaging. According to one patient, "If I do bring [a treatment] up, they'll say there is a waiting list, such as for an MRI [magnetic resonance imaging], so it will take longer, so by that time I would rather just suck it up rather than wait."

Just over one-quarter of patients (*n* = 15) did not report discussing treatment options with their providers, and about one-third (*n* = 17) felt that they were not offered a choice of treatments. Patients shared that sometimes this occurred because they had already tried all available treatment options for their pain, whereas others were just not made aware of treatment options. As one patient noted, "I was told that at this point with where I'm at, that really this was the only option available to me." Another stated, "I didn't know my options. I didn't know what I could or couldn't do. . . . It's just kind of—I could say my ignorance of not knowing how the medical field works—but it's also that they try to get you in and out as fast as possible." A patient explained,

> It always starts off with like, "Here is some type of Motrin or pain reliever I can take over the counter and then . . . here are these stretches you can try at home on your own time," and when I go back, "The next course of action we can try is physical therapy." The next step is cortisone injections, and after that, if I'm still going back, for last resort, [there is] some type of surgery. It normally takes a while before you get to that. I feel like . . . they try to alleviate [your pain by] trying to avoid doing anything additional in terms of [other treatment options for] pain.

Of those who were queried (*n* = 51), most patients (*n* = 33) responded that their providers adequately explained the risks and benefits of treatments. Patients described providers that explained the risks and benefits of a variety of treatments, such as surgery and physical therapy, by listing out the pros and cons. In doing so, one patient noted,

> [My provider] started with the risks first, [be]cause risks have more consequences than benefits and then, what could happen . . . and as in depth as he went with that, he [also] went in depth with all the good things that could come with physical therapy, occupational therapy, and training, and took his time [explaining].

Providers explained how patients' duties would be affected by certain treatments. For example, the long healing time from a surgery was framed as a risk, in addition to steroid injections disqualifying a service member from flying an aircraft. Patients felt that providers explaining the risks and benefits for treatment was also used to justify when they made treatment recommendations, "or why they think this is the best option." In many cases, if the patients felt that the benefits outweighed the risk, they were willing to try the treatment.

However, a little under a quarter of patients ($n = 12$) thought their providers inadequately explained the risks and benefits of a treatment. Most notably, patients mentioned that they were unaware of the risks their treatments posed, ranging from surgery healing time to medication side effects. As one patient explained, "I thought it would be 12 weeks and I'd be done. Having talked to a physical therapist now, he said it'll probably be a year postsurgery to when I'm back to normal. I don't think it was laid out for me." Similarly, another patient shared that he was unaware of the risks of rapid discontinuation of gabapentin:

> Right around Christmastime was when they put me on gabapentin [anticonvulsant]. And they didn't give me any refills and didn't tell me you're supposed to scale down [i.e., taper off the medication], which I did naturally because I saw that I was running low and I didn't want to stop [all of a sudden]. It seemed like it made sense to weeble wobble down. And then I came back [to be seen in the pain care clinic], and they were like, "You just stopped [taking gabapentin (anticonvulsant)]? That could cause some problems." And I asked, and they said, "Well, with the drugs, the big one [side effect] is grogginess in the morning but take that earlier in the morning." But that didn't get brought up [i.e., they did not explain the risk of stopping the medication without a taper], or all the other side effects. It was like, "I don't want to tell you all the one-off side effects, because of that thing where you think about it [a side effect] and make it happen."

When asked whether their providers recommended one type of treatment over another ($n = 50$), patient feedback was mixed; nearly half of these patients ($n = 24$) said that they did, and others ($n = 20$) said that they did not. Of those whose providers recommended a type of treatment, patients reported that their providers most commonly recommended NPT ($n = 12$); a smaller number received recommendations for medication ($n = 6$) or surgery or invasive procedures ($n = 4$). Patients reported that their providers tended to first recommend less-invasive treatments, most commonly physical therapy. Patients often reported that their providers would offer other treatments after NPT, such as injections, NSAID patches, and surgery. A patient explained,

> [The provider] recommended I do back classes [in physical therapy] and not stick to medication, because . . . she didn't want me to become reliant on it. . . . So she did want me to

go to the back class [in physical therapy], so I can figure it out for myself and not rely on the medication.

Of those who were asked about whether their providers listened to their treatment preferences (n = 53), most patients (n = 37) reported that their providers listened to their treatment preferences; fewer than one-fifth of patients (n = 9) did not feel this way. A patient described the decisionmaking process with their provider:

There wasn't much, "Hey, this is another option, and this is why it's better or worse." It was more, "Here's what I'm thinking of and here's the pros and cons of that one. And then we can go to the next step." Which makes sense to me because you're the doctor and the expert. So I can go with what you say.

As one patient explained, "I think we definitely have a shared decisionmaking process, right, where they explain certain things to me, and then they offer me one source of treatment. And I accept or deny."

The main reason patients did not feel listened to was related to limited time with providers. A patient stated, "When I came in, it was like a conveyor belt, they were trying to get as many people out as possible: treat, treat, treat, to get to the next person. It actually took multiple visits to get to something that helped." Another reported, "I had one [provider] who basically told me I had to do physical therapy and Motrin, what more do I want. And that was a military doctor." Furthermore, patients also focused on the importance of advocating for their treatment preferences. One explained,

It's more like, if you don't advocate, you're not getting it. For anything. Especially related to pain. Even medication, if you came in, they're like, here you go. You didn't ask my history to see if I've already been prescribed that. You don't get that until you tell them that I've tried that and didn't have a good history. You have to know medication to have them give it to you. And I don't want the good stuff. I don't want narcotics.

Another described the importance of researching ahead of time so providers would listen to their preferences:

Yes, like I said, the first time I was really trying to advocate. I don't know if it was an education thing, or just a reluctance to refer out to specialty care, given the limited assets, but again, once I hit the tipping point, when I asked for something, it was much easier to secure it.

Patient Perceptions of Treatment Options

Care for chronic pain includes a variety of treatments, including medication and NPT, such as physical therapy, acupuncture, and cognitive behavioral therapy. We asked patients (n = 54) to share their preferences or thoughts about different treatment options. In follow-up probes, patients were queried about whether they preferred NPT or medications, whether they had preferences for particular treatments, and whether they had any concerns about particular treatments. We also inquired about whether there was a treatment that a provider had recommended that the patient declined. Overall, most patients (n = 45) expressed some opinion about the treatments they preferred for chronic pain (e.g., treatments they wanted or treatments they preferred not to receive). However, even though most patients cited that they had preferences for their pain treatment options, a fraction (n = 9) did not endorse any preferences or stated they were willing to follow the treatment plan their providers recommended.

Over half of patients (n = 31) indicated that they preferred NPT. Some of these patients (n = 13) cited positive past experiences with NPT as a reason for their preferring it over medications. Additionally, many NPTs, such as physical therapy, are primarily patient-driven and rely on a combination of behavior change and education. Patients who appreciated physical therapy described it as a more active and empowering form of treatment, as they were able to work toward achieving their goals with each session, compared with passively having to take medication. A patient described the benefits of NPT by stating,

> At that point, it goes back to if an individual does not know [how to manage pain], another individual will teach you a better way on how to either deal with or handle your problems in a better manner, or at least teach you that, "Hey, I know you have this problem. We could improve on these aspects to strengthen that or reduce the problem." It's not going to cure the problem, but I always enjoyed the face-to-face interaction. . . . So that's my only preference when it comes down to getting the treatment: someone there to see what's wrong with me, identif[y] what's wrong with me, provide me these solutions, along with making sure that I'm doing it correctly.

Other patients (n = 11) preferred NPT because of their perceived effectiveness and lack of side effects, and some (n = 8) mentioned other reasons, including the self-directed nature of certain NPT, such as physical therapy.

The overarching consensus among those who preferred NPT was that they did not want to take medications for their pain treatment. When asked to elaborate on their preferences for particular treatments, some patients (n = 20) responded by describing the intervention that they preferred *not* to receive: medication. The most common reasons cited in explanation for this was the side effects of medication and a perceived lack of effectiveness (n = 12). Patients believed that medications led to adverse reactions or tolerance, and service members worried that this could negatively affect their duties. As one patient described,

> I think [medication is] just a Band-Aid, a placebo effect. . . . Obviously, if you have a cold, cold medicine can help you out, but I just look at elderly people who are taking a bunch of medications to benefit their life, because you know they have knee pain, or low back pain, or whatever case may be, and eventually, their low-dosage medication isn't working anymore because their body has built up a tolerance to it, to where they need a higher milligram [dosage]. Ultimately, your body can't process that; you're taking liver pills to

help you function. So, I'm all for medication, but as long as there's an end point to it. Not necessarily: This is what I gotta take for the rest of my life.

Another patient (aged 35 to 44 years) stated:

> A lot of my compatriots would benefit more from doing an active medical recovery rather than a prescribed one. . . . And I understand that's maybe not the focus, but I can probably count on two hands the number of people I know that are no longer here, because they succumbed to [opioid] prescription overdose. And so it's something that me and my generation of service members have kind of, not sworn off, but we're kind of reticent to participate in when it comes to prescription medications. . . . We prefer to do treatments, you know, with a specialist or doing some sort of activity or doing a collective event that facilitates recovery. And that's just the trend within my generation of folks.

Another patient reported, "I would say that the physical therapy and the sports medicine and . . . the nonprescription treatments [are beneficial]. I've witnessed others participate in [those and] were more successful and got after the root causes faster and more succinctly than just writing another prescription."

In contrast, a handful of patients ($n = 6$) stated that they preferred receiving medication over NPT. These patients cited lower time commitment with medications compared with NPT, among other reasons. One patient reported that he liked taking medication because of the ease of taking it whenever he wanted to, compared with commuting an hour to an NPT appointment, paying for gas prices, and losing the day to the appointment. Another mentioned that he was interested in the idea of physical therapy, but because of his duties as a senior officer, had trouble finding a convenient time to attend appointments. Another service member mentioned the positive experience he had with the cannabinoid Marinol with reducing his pain. Others ($n = 5$) indicated that they preferred receiving other treatments, such as injections or surgery, over medication or NPT, versus several patients ($n = 4$) who preferred *not* to receive injections or surgery.

Among patients who answered our probe about whether they had concerns about particular treatments ($n = 48$), nearly half ($n = 23$) did not have any concerns. Among those who did have concerns about treatments ($n = 25$), many of the themes overlapped with those we heard with respect to patient treatment preferences. For example, over one-quarter of patients ($n = 17$) stated or reiterated that they had concerns about medication, with many citing medication side effects or lack of effectiveness as the primary reason. Several patients ($n = 5$) expressed concern about a specific NPT, typically based on their past experience with the treatment not being effective. Other patients ($n = 6$) expressed general concerns about treatment, such as perceiving their treatment plan not to be effective or worrying about the possibility of reinjury or the need for surgery.

Finally, we asked most patients ($n = 50$) whether they declined any treatments that their providers recommended. Most ($n = 31$) reported that there were no treatments they declined.

Those who declined a treatment (n = 20) reported declining medication (n = 9), NPT (n = 8), or surgery (n = 6); two patients stated that they had declined more than one treatment.

Treatment Adjustment

In this section, we discuss themes related to provider views on factors considered in treatment adjustment and patient perspectives on treatment adjustment.

Factors Considered by Providers in Treatment Adjustment

We asked providers (n = 53) about factors that they considered in making the determination of whether and how to adjust a patient's treatment for chronic pain. Although we did not probe for specific patient, treatment, and organizational factors considered, we coded and summarized themes in that format. Overall, the most common factors that providers considered in treatment adjustment were the pain severity or impact on patient functioning and treatment effectiveness.

Nearly all providers (n = 50) cited the importance of assessing the severity of pain symptoms or the impact of the chronic pain condition on patient functioning. In discussing this consideration, providers mentioned the use of structured assessment tools, such as the DVPRS or PASTOR, or described using unstructured questioning to inquire about the impact of pain on patients' daily activities. As one provider explained, "We use the pain scale to see where [patients] are at with their pain, and how they manage it day to day, and if it impacts their activities or duty at work. And if it does, then we will look to make modifications at that point." Another stated, "I'll kind of just ask subjectively how they [patients] think about how [treatment is] going. What limitations they have, what things would they like to be able to do that they aren't able to do." Relatedly, one-quarter of providers (n = 14) identified service member duties, responsibilities, or career as a consideration in treatment adjustment. One provider shared, "I look mainly to see [whether patients are] able to perform all duties of their MOS. Are they able to do different components of the physical fitness test?" Other providers described assessing functional impairment to determine the need for a limited-duty profile or to determine implications for the patient's military career. As one provider stated, "I also try to consider their active-duty status, if they had duty restrictions like light or limited duty, and then they have a certain amount of time they can be on those restrictions. So obviously if they are running out of time, then I will maybe speed up their [treatment]." Additionally, some providers (n = 10) discussed considering patient preferences or perceptions in approaching treatment adjustment (e.g., patient satisfaction with degree of improvement in pain symptoms), and some (n = 7) stated that they would consider the success of past treatments received before making any changes. Some providers (n = 5) also cited other patient-related considerations, including the frequency of refill requests or the number of follow-up visits needed to address a patient's pain care. We provide further detail on provider perspectives of assessment of the impact of pain on functioning later in this chapter.

Treatment effectiveness was mentioned by most respondents ($n = 37$) across all MTFs as an important factor in assessing the need for an adjustment. As with provider remarks about pain symptoms and patient functioning, treatment effectiveness was typically discussed in the context of a structured or unstructured assessment of pain. As one provider shared,

> If they're moving toward getting better, then we'll say, "This medication seems to be working." If they're not making progress or [if they're moving in the] wrong direction . . . I'll say, "What are some other [treatments] that you'd like to try?"

Some providers ($n = 8$) also mentioned assessing a patient's tolerance of the treatment, including side effects. One provider mentioned CPGs or clinic treatment policies concerning treatment adjustment.

Patient Perception of Treatment Adjustment

For some patients, pain treatment can involve making changes to treatment or trying different treatments. Examples of these are changes in the dose or the type of medication or trying a non-medication treatment, such as physical therapy. We asked patients whether they had received any treatment adjustment in the past six months ($n = 54$). Some patients ($n = 18$) said that they had not. Over half of patients ($n = 36$) had received a treatment adjustment. Among those who did, most patients ($n = 22$) reported a medication change, such as a change in dose or stopping or changing medication. Fewer patients ($n = 12$) described trying an NPT or changing an NPT. Several patients ($n = 5$) described another type of treatment change, such as referrals to orthopedic or sports medicine. The most common reason for treatment adjustment among patients ($n = 24$) was the persistence of pain despite treatment. Other patients spoke of wanting a treatment change that would provide pain relief and improve their quality of life, help return them to normal activities, and become a "functional member of my community right now." Certain patients reported multiple clinic visits for treatment adjustments:

> It was more of me going and going and going, bothering them so they can get tired of me. Because I needed help with back pain. It bothers me while driving, sitting, watching TV, walking. I used to be active, work out a lot, run a lot, and now my soldiers run past me. I wanted to get back to what I was."

Patients highlighted the importance of advocating for themselves to get a treatment adjustment:

> Yeah [I was the one needing to advocate] because in the military they get you in and out as fast as possible because they've got everyone coming in. So, they were trying to just see what the limit of it could be and go to that. Do the bare minimum to get you out and working.

Finally, patients who experienced a treatment adjustment ($n = 36$) were queried on whether providers used their understanding of pain's impact on their functioning to make the adjustment. Most of those patients ($n = 24$) responded positively, indicating that providers did use pain impact on the patient's daily activities to change treatment, although other patients ($n = 11$) did not. Patients described their providers recommending treatment based on reading the patient's medical record, understanding their work duties, and discussing their pain symptoms. These patients reported high levels of shared decisionmaking, which was generally well received. However, one patient commented about the drawbacks of patients driving treatment adjustments, stating,

> They defer to me and let me decide [the course of treatment]. But this is your profession. If they are easily swayed by the patient, that is sometimes a good thing, sometimes a bad thing. Sometimes I might be making the wrong call [about treatment]. I don't think they look at the impact [of my pain] on my daily life and think, "Oh gosh, I am not getting better." I think it's like, "Okay she's happy, she's out the door." I think I might be the cause of it.

Some patients felt that their providers did not consider the impact of their pain on their daily activities ($n = 11$). These patients felt that their providers still tried to manage their pain, but the takeaway often was, "You're going to be dealing with pain; we'll try to keep it as low as we can" or "It's going to affect you, so learn to live with it and mitigate it." We provide further detail on patients' perspectives on the assessment of the impact of pain on their functioning later in this chapter.

Assessment of Pain's Impact on Functioning

In this section, we summarize provider and patient perspectives on the assessment of pain's impact on functioning.

Provider Perceptions of Assessment of Pain's Impact on Functioning

We asked all providers ($n = 53$) how they assessed how pain affected a patient's daily activities among service members with chronic pain. Nearly all providers ($n = 51$) across all MTFs told us that they used some method for this purpose; slightly more than half ($n = 27$) reported use of a structured assessment, such as the DVPRS or PASTOR, and slightly less than half ($n = 24$) described an unstructured method of asking questions to determine patient functioning. Among those who endorsed using a structured approach, the DVPRS was the most common tool: Some providers ($n = 17$) referenced the DVPRS specifically, whereas others ($n = 7$) described an unspecified rating scale in their EHR system that prompted patients to give a pain rating on a scale of 1 to 10, followed by questions about how pain affects functioning for patients with scores of 4 or higher. As one provider shared,

So, like the DVPRS scale is a helpful tool. That just helps us to see how the patient is functioning, especially over time. And just how they're feeling. What their level of function is, if they're able to maintain their job, if they feel like they're getting worse, better, or staying the same. That's the main thing, just seeing how they're functioning. And that will help us guide their treatment.

Additionally, some providers ($n = 7$), all of whom worked in an MTF pain clinic, described using PASTOR, a more in-depth assessment and follow-up tool, to examine changes in patient-reported functioning over time. Several of the respondents who used the DVPRS or PASTOR described working with medical technicians or other team members to ensure the regular administration of these assessments. In contrast, among the respondents who used unstructured methods of pain assessment ($n = 24$), most asked questions during the visit to assess for patient functioning and improvement. As one provider shared,

I look mainly to see, are they able to perform all duties of their MOS? Are they able to do different components of the physical fitness test? Is the pain impeding on other lifestyle things? . . . If they are having difficulties with any of those things, reassessing where we are with treatments."

Patient Perceptions of Assessment of Pain's Impact on Functioning

We asked all patients ($n = 54$) whether, over the past six months, their provider evaluated the impact of their pain on their daily activities. Nearly all patients ($n = 52$) affirmed that providers had performed a pain assessment. Of those patients, about half ($n = 25$) said that providers used a structured or survey-based method, such as a questionnaire or pain scale. One patient remarked, "[They asked] how I'm doing, on a pain scale 1 to 10. Then they kind of picked up from where we left off at the last session, on my abilities and what I was able to do. [For example], have I progressed or regressed? Very thorough." Only a few patients ($n = 3$) felt that their providers did not assess the impact of pain on their daily activities. One patient described how, in their experience, it was usually self-initiated:

Trying to find out the level of impact to my daily activities is not [something that was asked]. I can't remember having that question or that discussion. Normally I'm the one who initiates that because I do know that I don't often get asked those questions [about how pain affects me and my daily activities]. But I try to insert that into the discussion, just to make the providers aware that my pain is not only me experiencing pain. It is also impacting either my professional life or social life.

Among the patients specifically asked about the frequency of pain assessment ($n = 49$), most ($n = 34$) indicated that they were asked during every visit, whereas others ($n = 6$) reported they were asked most visits, and other patients ($n = 6$) were asked rarely. For patients asked about which providers performed an assessment of pain and its impact on functioning

(n = 46), many (n = 31) stated that all or most of their providers asked about how pain affects their daily activities, whereas other patients (n = 7) said that some (e.g., half of) providers did, and several (n = 4) indicated that few or no providers asked. One patient indicated that pain assessment was variable between providers. Physical therapy was a commonly mentioned setting where providers conducted pain assessments.

Patient Perceptions of Coordination of Care

Coordination of care includes a variety of activities from providers reading the notes from other providers in a patient's medical record to communicating directly with different providers about a patient's care. We asked patients who had more than one provider treating their pain at the same time (n = 46) whether their providers communicated well with each other about their care. Some of these patients (n = 17) reported that providers had communicated well, and we asked them to elaborate on what indicated that there had been good provider-provider communication. On the other hand, some patients (n = 17) said that their providers did not communicate well with each other. Other patients (n = 7) gave variable responses, indicating that some providers communicated whereas others did not. Several patients (n = 5) were unsure or did not offer an opinion about whether their providers communicated with one another about their pain care.

Patients Who Reported That Their Providers Communicated Well

Among those patients who reported that their providers communicated well with one another about patient care (n = 17), a majority believed that their providers were actively reading each other's notes in the medical record (n = 14). One explained, "I do get the sense that [my provider] does check my record. . . . I'll walk in, and he'll ask me about something I've complained about in the past. Like the physical therapy, there was a lapse with that guy, but he's got his notes, and he'll check his notes." Another noted,

> [The doctor] . . . takes time to read some of the notes, and then he'll say, "okay, I see you've mentioned this, that, and the other, is that correct?" And I agree or deny. And most of the time, it's agreeing. And that leads me to believe that the records are accurate and detailed.

Patients also commented on the value of detailed notes in the medical record to support provider communication. In some cases, that made care transition easier and seamless. According to one patient,

> [The providers are] good [at communicating] because one provider was pregnant when I was seeing her and she had her baby, so she was out for a few months. The detailed notes she left in my record—the next provider was able to see it. I only saw him once, and their long-term physical therapist showed up and I've seen him. He has all the detailed notes, so it's been a lot smoother than it normally would have been.

Other patients who said their providers communicated well with one another elaborated by citing evidence of the providers speaking directly to coordinate care ($n = 8$). This more effective level of communication between providers was most evident in MTF pain clinics. One patient explained,

> So, at the pain clinic it seems like they all know each other. And the fact that they openly talk to one another like on a normal basis, when you're going from one person to the next. It's almost . . . like everybody knows, like, "Hey, you know we've tried this, like what do you think about this? I know this doctor would agree, I'm going to talk to this [provider] first." [It's] pretty nice being able to have a whole team pretty much looking after you, although they might work in like separate areas. It's like one tiny little community [in the pain management clinic], pretty much.

A few patients ($n = 3$) said that their providers simply "seemed to know" about care the patient received through another clinic or provider.

Patients Who Reported That Their Providers Did Not Communicate Well

Among patients who stated that providers did not communicate well ($n = 17$), various explanations were provided. In some cases, these patients understood that providers read each other's notes but did not feel this was sufficient communication, and described being asked questions that were already answered in the medical record. There were also instances of communication breakdowns in which patients received separate directions from two different providers. One explained,

> No, I don't think [my providers] communicated ever. I received two different sets of directions [from the PCM and physical therapist]; it was kinda hard to know who to follow. [The] physical therapist—[they're] trained in this, [so] do I do [what they say]? And then I would go to physical therapy and follow up with my PCM, and then I might get, "You don't need to do that." Well, that's what the [physical therapist] said. There seems to be conflict in terms of care.

Additionally, patients experienced instances of referral outcomes falling through because of a lack of care coordination. Patients reported instances in which the provider who made the referral for an imaging test never followed up with them, and they reached out themselves to find out the results. One patient stated, "In certain instances, what I always heard was, 'Yeah, you should have been informed about this. I don't know why it didn't happen,' and stuff like that. So, I've had this actually happen a couple times."

Patients Who Reported That Communication Between Providers Was Variable

Other patients ($n = 7$) felt that care coordination and communication varied between providers at different settings, stating that some of their providers communicated with one another whereas others did not. These patients also had more-mixed responses about adequacy of communication in cases when it had occurred. For example, one patient reported that their primary care provider tended not to communicate well with other providers but stated, "physical therapy was on top of it [communication], and the specialty care, they were actually on top of it also. They knew the information before I got in there and they confirmed what the report said and what I had said and went from there." A few of these patients citing variable communication said that this level of communication was inadequate ($n = 2$). For example, one patient remarked, "I would love to see more communication. I think any time when there is a group [of] professionals that are talking, there's a lot of good things that can happen. It would also make me feel like I'm receiving more-comprehensive care." Other patients citing variable communication did not comment on whether they felt that this level of communication was adequate ($n = 5$).

Patient Perceptions of Treatment Equity

MTFs provide pain care for service members from many different backgrounds. We asked patients ($n = 54$) whether they felt they had been treated differently during their pain care because of some aspect of their background, such as age, race and ethnicity, gender, rank, sexual identity and orientation, religion, and income. About three-quarters of respondents ($n = 41$) indicated that they had not been treated differently, whereas nearly one-quarter ($n = 12$) felt as though they had been treated differently because of their background. One person was unsure whether they had been treated differently, remarking, "I try not to think of that, it shouldn't matter."

Of those who reported that they had been treated differently ($n = 12$), most ($n = 8$) described receiving unfavorable treatment, whereas the remainder ($n = 4$) reported receiving preferential treatment on the basis of rank or military occupation. Although respondents could be included in more than one category, the most common reason for feeling as though they had been treated unfavorably was because of rank or age ($n = 4$). One patient indicated that they had been treated differently because of their military occupation. Other reasons mentioned included gender ($n = 1$), race and ethnicity ($n = 1$), and the perception of receiving unfair treatment because of favoritism shown toward other patients ($n = 1$). Two patients believed that they were treated negatively but did not provide a specific reason ($n = 2$). When patients spoke of being treated unfavorably because of age and rank, they reported seeing higher-ranking service members getting more-timely treatments. A patient explained, "I've seen higher-ranking [service members] with similar issues get treated almost immediately after they go in there. And then the junior ranking, they don't get treated as quickly, and [providers] try to beat around the bush with it." Another commented, "Just from sitting in the [clinic] lobby, certain people take precedence over others, in terms of rank, or the buddy system [i.e., favoritism]." Some also spoke of using their connections to navigate the military health system to overcome obstacles and receive care and how access to care differed based on unit. For example, the walk-in hours at clinics for some units were shorter compared with other units, limiting access and availability of services.

A patient commented on age and how he perceived it affecting his treatment:

> I think me being only 26 with the back issues that I have, I have maybe once or twice have not been taken as seriously. But that's just verbally. . . . there have just been a few interactions with people of, "You really have this bad of a back issue? You're only 26." But it was nothing that really bothered me, I still have gotten the care.

In a similar light, another patient spoke of not being taken seriously because of her age and gender:

> I just remember feeling like they weren't taking me seriously because I'm really young first of all and I'm small. I'm a female. So, I couldn't have been through that much to make me need stuff, so that's one of the things, yeah. So, I feel like they didn't care enough to look into something more.

The same patient commented that she felt that female providers acknowledged her pain more and were more thorough with her pain treatment compared with male providers; she shared that male providers only prescribed NSAIDs and did not ask any further questions.

A patient also detailed an instance in which their pain treatment and options differed from a coworker because of race:

> I have a coworker who also goes to [the] physical therapy clinic and she's the same rank and female, but she's white. She'll come back [after her appointment] and say, "They referred me and we're going to do all of these things." And I'm like, "Huh, okay, I didn't get those options, I wonder why." We both have an ortho, knee injury, that affects the hip and back, the same kind of issue, but a different course of action [has] been taken with the both of us.

Another patient emphasized that although their providers were well-intentioned, the patient had experienced gaps in care:

> No, I don't think so [that I have been treated differently]. . . . I think the providers we have, at least the ones I've dealt with, I think they mean well. I think they care about providing the best care possible to our service members. But then again . . . there have been noticeable [gaps], like the ones I just mentioned about not really discussing what those impacts [of pain] are to my professional or social life, or not following up with the notes or the results of imaging or lab work. So those were the gaps that I have noticed. But other than that, I don't think there's a willful or malicious intent on the part of our providers.

Among those who described receiving favorable treatment ($n = 4$), military occupation or advanced rank was cited as the reason for preferential treatment. For example, a patient spoke of being treated differently in a positive way because of a higher rank:

> I know I get different treatment now, however, based on my experience from years ago when I wasn't a "somebody" here [at the hospital], I'm not offered different treatments, but being a senior officer, I'm probably not pushed as hard as they would a younger soldier because I'm at the end of my career and it won't affect my long-term career options. Whereas if they were worried about me achieving on the physical readiness test, I'm going, "I can do that test lying down, even with a broken back, and I'm retiring in a few years." The answer is, yeah, I get treated differently, but not in a negative way.

Another patient remarked,

> The older, more senior, more assertive, the person is, the more experienced [they are], [the providers are going to] take care of him a certain way. It's a psychological response. . . . Fifteen years in [to my military service], especially [after being] deployed the [majority of the] amount of time, [providers tend to take me more seriously].

Patients who stated that they had not been treated differently ($n = 41$) generally gave more definitive responses. For example, one patient said, "I don't think I've been discriminated [against]. I don't think so." Numerous patients responded with, "No, not at all," and another patient remarked, "No, not that I've experienced." Thus, although a majority of service members felt that they were not treated differently because of their background, there were some instances in which that was not the case.

Summary

In this chapter, we described themes from interviews with providers and patients related to treatment planning and adjustment and the assessment of pain's impact on functioning. We also presented findings from patient interviews with respect to care coordination and equity.

- **Treatment planning and shared decisionmaking:** With respect to factors considered by providers in treatment planning, the availability of treatments (or lack thereof) and the type, severity, duration, or impact of the patient's pain condition were the most common considerations. Half of providers also described service member duties, patient preference, and other patient-related factors (e.g., age, diet, and lifestyle) as important considerations. Nearly all providers endorsed the idea that the patient plays a role in the treatment planning process, and about half of these interviewees endorsed each of the following themes: building patient buy-in, providing patients with treatment options, and determining the interests or goals of the patient with respect to treatment options. Relatedly, most patients said that they were offered a choice of treatment options, felt that their providers explained the benefits and risks of treatments, and believed that their providers listened to their preferences for treatment. Regarding preferences for the treatment of chronic pain, over half of all patients said that they preferred NPT, and it was the most frequently offered treatment.

- **Treatment adjustment and pain assessment:** The most common consideration in treatment adjustment mentioned by nearly all providers was the assessment of the severity of pain symptoms or the impact of the pain condition on patient functioning. Slightly more than half of all providers reported that they used a structured method, such as the DVPRS or PASTOR, to assess the impact of pain on functioning. This objective outcome measurement is consistent with the stepped-care model, which aims for a patient's return to functioning, with care adjusted to patient needs over time. Nearly all patients reported that their treatment had been adjusted in some way in the past six months; most cited a lack of adequate treatment response or improvement as the reason for the adjustment. Themes from patient interviews with respect to assessment were consistent with those from providers; most patients reported that one or more providers assessed the impact of their pain on their daily activities in some way (i.e., through unstructured or structured means). When asked, most patients reported that these assessments were administered at every visit and by all or most of their pain care providers. Among the patients whose treatment had been adjusted within the past six months, most felt that their provider had used their understanding of the impact of pain on their daily activities to make the adjustment. These findings support the implementation of stepped care (e.g., NPT before more-invasive treatment) and regular assessment of patient response and functioning as a basis for treatment adjustment.
- **Care coordination and equity:** Fewer than half of patients who had more than one provider treating their pain at the same time reported that providers communicated well with one another about their care. Patients who felt that their providers communicated well believed that their providers were reviewing medical record documentation by other providers or that their providers were communicating with each other directly. A similar number of patients felt that their providers did not communicate well with each other about their pain care. They cited incidents of lack of coordination, such as being given conflicting treatment recommendations, or a lack of follow-up on treatment results. Most patients felt that they had been treated equitably, but nearly one-quarter of patients felt they had been treated differently because of their background. The most common reasons patients believed that they were treated differently were related to age and rank.

CHAPTER 5

Pharmacologic Treatment for Chronic Pain

In this chapter, we describe themes on pharmacologic treatment for chronic pain from interviews with providers, administrators, and patients. Chronic pain medications include NSAIDs, non-NSAID analgesics, anticonvulsants, muscle relaxants, antidepressants, and opioids. Medications may be administered orally, topically, or by injection. The MHS stepped-care model for pain care encourages treatment with NPT or nonopioid medication and minimizes the use of opioids (Defense Health Agency Procedural Instruction 6025.04, 2018). Here, we describe factors considered by providers when prescribing opioids and administrator views on processes to support providers in appropriate opioid prescribing. We also discuss the barriers faced by providers and administrators with respect to providing opioid medication treatments for chronic pain. Next, we discuss nonopioid medications most often used by providers to treat service members with chronic pain. Additionally, we describe patient experiences with medications received for pain in the past six months.

Prescriber Perspectives on Opioid Prescribing

In this section, we present findings on prescriber perspectives on factors considered in opioid prescribing for chronic pain. As discussed in Chapter 2, we asked providers ($n = 53$) to respond to structured questions indicating whether they were providing opioid medication treatment to or managing long-term opioid use for service members at the time of their interview (see Table 2.4). Of the providers who were licensed to prescribe medications (hereafter referred to as *prescribers*; $n = 50$), all reported that prescribing opioid medications would be consistent with their scope of clinical practice. However, some prescribers ($n = 9$) indicated that they were not providing opioid medication treatment (of any duration) to service members, and half of all prescribers ($n = 25$) said that they were prescribing opioids but were not managing service members with chronic pain on LOT. Despite this variation in prescribing practices, all prescribers discussed the factors that they considered in prescribing opioids for chronic pain, even if they were not currently providing opioids for chronic pain to service members at their MTF. In the next section, we summarize the views of all prescribers ($n = 50$) with respect to opioid prescribing to treat service members with chronic pain.

Factors Considered by Prescribers in Opioid Prescribing

We asked all prescribers, including those who were not currently prescribing opioids to service members, about factors that influenced whether they would prescribe an opioid to a service member with chronic pain ($n = 50$). In our follow-up probes, we prompted prescribers to consider the role of patient factors (e.g., patient presentation or preferences), provider or treatment factors (e.g., provider preferences and treatment effectiveness), and structural or organizational factors (e.g., factors related to clinic operations, policies, or programs). Thematic differences emerged in prescriber responses based on their stated comfort level with opioid prescribing in general: Prescribers who expressed trepidation about opioid prescribing ($n = 45$) generally discussed different considerations than did prescribers who said they would prescribe opioids to service members with chronic pain when clinically appropriate to do so ($n = 5$). In this section, we summarize themes separately for these two groups.

Factors Considered by Prescribers Who Expressed Reluctance About Opioid Prescribing

Nearly all prescribers across all MTFs expressed reluctance about opioid prescribing for chronic pain ($n = 45$). Despite their trepidation, most of these individuals ($n = 36$) stated that they were currently prescribing opioids (for any duration) to one or more service members, and about half ($n = 22$) said that they were currently managing one or more service members with chronic pain on LOT. A fraction of these reluctant prescribers ($n = 6$) also mentioned in the interview that opioids were among the medications that they used the most to treat service members with chronic pain.

Regardless of whether they were currently providing opioid treatment, providers expressed reluctance with respect to prescribing opioids. Most of these individuals ($n = 37$) told us that they rarely or never initiate a prescription for opioids to active-duty service members with chronic pain, whereas the remainder ($n = 8$) said that they would consider prescribing but only as a last resort. Among those who would rarely or never initiate opioid prescriptions for chronic pain ($n = 37$), their remarks about prescribing practices were varied. Some ($n = 11$) mentioned that they would attempt to taper inherited LOT patients off opioids, whereas some ($n = 9$) said that they would consider prescribing an opioid for chronic pain to *bridge* or maintain an existing opioid prescription initiated by another prescriber. Some of these reluctant prescribers who rarely or never initiated opioid medication treatment for chronic pain ($n = 8$) said that they would consider prescribing opioids for acute exacerbations of chronic pain but not for a longer duration. A few ($n = 3$) said that they would simply never prescribe opioids.

Over half of all prescribers who expressed reluctance about opioid prescribing for chronic pain ($n = 30$) expressed concern about the addiction potential of opioids, side effects, or safety. As one respondent stated, "It's a slippery slope with opioids, because of their addictive properties. . . . You know, there's an opioid crisis going on. I think Netflix even recently did a documentary on it." Another reported,

Chronic pain, I don't do it [prescribe opioids]. Unless they've already been on the opioid. And even if they are, let's say I have a patient, my patients know I don't prescribe opioids, and that's something your panel will learn. But if I get a new patient that is on opioids, I will do my damnedest to find another provider in the clinic that prescribes opioids to have them see them. If I can't, I will do a bridge until they can be seen by either a specialist or their PCM.

Some of these reluctant prescribers ($n = 16$) expressed concern about deployment readiness or reported that prescribing opioids for more than a short period would result in medical separation from the military. Others ($n = 18$) felt that opioids were not effective for chronic pain or that other treatments were equally or more effective. About one-quarter ($n = 12$) said that they were uncomfortable or inexperienced with opioid prescribing for chronic pain. Other themes included clinic or MTF culture (e.g., "I can tell you nobody probably in my clinic has started somebody on an opioid") ($n = 7$), the time-consuming burden of managing opioid oversight requirements ("It is cumbersome [prescribing opioids]; it does require more monitoring") ($n = 9$), and medical training or past professional experience (e.g., "I think when I was in residency and kind of getting my training through this whole quote unquote opioid epidemic, I have a pretty negative association of opioids") ($n = 5$). Explained one provider,

[Prescribers] just give people opiates because it's way easier than seeing them or weaning them off opiates. There is no time. No time in MTF schedule. You cannot see chronic pain patients in less than 15 minutes, which is what the MHS expects you to do. And pain monitoring—I have patients weaning off opiates and they're buying them from another provider across the MTF because someone is writing them a prescription for 120 opiates per month. So, I think getting all providers to hold the line is important. Because patients know who those providers are.

Factors Considered by Prescribers Who Were Willing to Prescribe Opioids for Chronic Pain

Several prescribers ($n = 5$) stated that they were willing to prescribe opioids to service members with chronic pain without endorsing reluctance or concern. All of these individuals ($n = 5$) were currently prescribing opioids, and the majority ($n = 3$) were currently managing service members on LOT at the time of the interview. The remainder of these more willing prescribers ($n = 2$) also mentioned in the interview that opioids were among the medications they used the most to treat service members with chronic pain.

Among this small cohort of prescribers who did not express reluctance about opioid prescribing for service members with chronic pain, all considered patient-related factors (e.g., pain condition type, severity, and impact on functioning) and organizational or structural factors (e.g., care coordination supports, the availability of consultation with a pain clinic specialist or pharmacist, and opioid prescribing feedback) in their approach to opioid prescribing for service members with chronic pain. One mentioned treatment-related factors, such as CPGs, and one mentioned provider-related factors, such as personal beliefs or professional training.

Processes to Support Providers in Prescribing Opioids

In this section, we present findings on administrator perspectives on processes to support providers in appropriate opioid prescribing. We asked administrators (n = 15) whether there were any processes in place to support providers in appropriately prescribing opioids for chronic pain, such as provider education, ongoing monitoring, or feedback.[1] Apart from providing these examples, we did not follow up with any specific probes. All administrators indicated that their MTF had one or more processes in place to support providers in prescribing opioids for chronic pain, citing a variety of different supports (Figure 5.1).[2] The most common of these, endorsed by most administrators across nearly all MTFs, was the availability of prescription monitoring feedback (n = 12). Additionally, most administrators (n = 10) across all MTFs discussed the availability of provider training on opioid prescribing, most (n = 9) mentioned the availability of consultation with a pain specialist or pain champion, and half (n = 8) mentioned the availability of pharmacist support for opioid prescribing. In the sections that follow, we provide additional detail on the supports that administrators discussed.

Prescription Monitoring Feedback to Support Opioid Prescribing

Over three-quarters of administrators (n = 12) across nearly all MTFs mentioned the availability of prescription monitoring feedback. Respondents described numerous different metrics in these monitoring feedback programs.[3] However, we did not ask respondents to indicate whether specific metrics were being monitored, and it may be that some respondents provided more-exhaustive responses than others. Metrics included the co-prescribing of naloxone (n = 7); establishing of sole prescriber contracts with patients (n = 6); avoiding the co-prescribing of benzodiazepines (n = 3); monitoring to encourage the lowest appropriate dose or MEDD (n = 4); conducting overdose risk assessments, such as computing the Risk Index for Overdose or Serious Opioid-Induced Respiratory Depression (RIOSORD) score (n = 2);

---

[1] Elsewhere, we summarize administrator-reported supports for provider use of NPT (Chapter 6) and staff-reported overarching facilitators of good pain care (Chapter 7).

[2] The MHS has a Prescription Drug Monitoring Program for centralized tracking of controlled substances prescribed to service members. In addition, the CarePoint MHS Opioid Registry provides decision support tools, such as calculated risk scores for opioid overdose. Some respondents specifically mentioned these tools in their responses, whereas others did not.

[3] MHS monitors prescriptions of 50 MME per day or higher, co-prescribing of benzodiazepines and opioids, the number of patients receiving LOT, and the receipt of naloxone for patients deemed high risk (U.S. Department of Defense, 2021).

FIGURE 5.1

Administrator-Reported Supports for Appropriate Opioid Prescribing

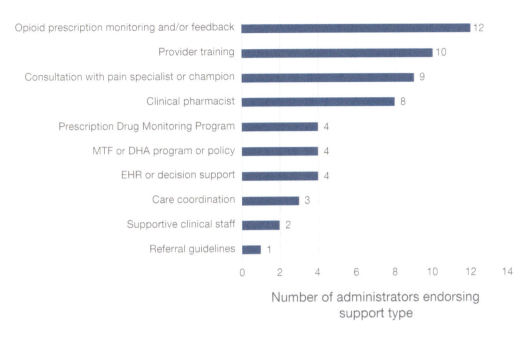

Number of administrators endorsing
support type

NOTE: Administrator-reported supports specific to the use of NPT and staff-reported overarching facilitators of good pain care are excluded from this figure; they are discussed in Chapters 6 and 7, respectively. $N = 15$.

and regular urine drug toxicology screening ($n = 2$). For example, as one administrator from a pain management clinic explained,

> We do a quarterly peer review. . . . Our pain pharmacist sadly just left us, but [for clinicians prescribing opioids,] quality control on distributing naloxone now . . . [is that] our nurse case manager goes through the records and makes sure everyone is in compliance in terms of urine drug screening and continuous monitoring for patients on chronic opioid therapy.

Another administrator from a pain management clinic in a different service branch described the monitoring activities conducted by the Long-Term Opioid Therapy Safety program at their MTF, stating,

> There are separate criteria to check and monitor at each visit: prescription drug monitoring, narcotics [prescribed by providers from] other places, concern from [risk of] diversion, are they getting benefit from meds [opioids] still, what is their functional status? These are things we are supposed to be checking. Calculating the RIOSORD score, or what their morphine equivalent daily dose is, to see if they qualify for naloxone.

Of the administrators who mentioned prescription monitoring feedback or support (n = 12), some (n = 7) also discussed the importance of using of CPGs to guide opioid prescribing. Some of the administrators also discussed how those feedback programs were facilitated through EHR or decision support tools (e.g., "red flag alerts based on morphine equivalents [or] number of prescribers") (n = 4), supportive MTF or clinic processes (e.g., central MTF oversight of pain care in primary care clinics) (n = 4), the use of a prescription drug monitoring database (n = 5), and the availability of nursing or ancillary staff to facilitate appropriate opioid prescribing (n = 2).

Provider Training on Appropriate Opioid Prescribing

Another common process mentioned by most administrators (n = 10) across nearly all MTFs, regardless of having formal prescription monitoring or support programs, was provider training on opioid prescribing. In some cases, training took the form of a DHA course or a curriculum prepared by a pain champion at the MTF. As one administrator explained, "We all have mandated opioid training we have to take. I want to say that's every two or three years? . . . That is mandated by DHA, is my understanding." In other cases, administrators mentioned that providers completed training on pain care as a part of their professional state licensure.

Consultation with a Pain Specialist or Pain Champion

Most administrators (n = 9) across nearly all MTFs mentioned the availability of consultation with a pain specialist or pain champion. Administrators at two MTFs mentioned Project ECHO as a resource for providers, either as a means of educating them directly or as a training resource for pain champions and a resource for MTF providers on opioid prescribing. One administrator explained, "We help facilitate the weekly ECHO, which is community outreach education. The primary audience is primary care pain champions. . . . They have a dedicated slot available [to attend meetings]." Other administrators described grand rounds or other clinic meetings as opportunities for providers to consult with pain champions or fellow providers on appropriate opioid prescribing. Explained one administrator, "A huge component of the curriculum that's pushed through our pain champion is just opioid education and management. He also does a screening tool through the pharmacy to pull patients that are on chronic opioids."

Pharmacist Support for Opioid Prescribing

Half of all administrators (n = 8) across most MTFs (representing all service branches) mentioned the availability of pharmacist support for opioid prescribing. All these individuals also reported having opioid prescribing monitoring programs at their respective clinics or MTFs. One administrator explained how clinical pharmacists were involved in providing feedback to providers, stating, "That's part of the pharmacists' [responsibilities]; they're required to check on opioids and will be alerted when patients are receiving opioids from multiple services. And [pharmacists] will let the PCMs know so that they receive that information." In addition to being involved in opioid prescribing monitoring programs, pharmacists were also consulted by individual providers to answer questions about prescribing or to assist with medication tapers. Said one administrator, "[Providers] can always go to the clinical pharmacist, and she is very knowledgeable. Just to troubleshoot and see what's best for the patient." In other cases, administrators described clinical pharmacists as being involved in provider education or dissemination of DHA guidance on opioid prescribing.

Other Supports for Opioid Prescribing

In addition to prescription monitoring and provider training, a few administrators also described care coordination (e.g., meetings at which providers discuss treatment for active-duty service members receiving LOT) ($n = 3$), the availability of nursing or ancillary staff (e.g., "our nurse case manager goes through the records and makes sure everyone is in compliance in terms of urine drug screening and continuous monitoring for patients on chronic opioid therapy") ($n = 2$), and helpful referral practices (e.g., guidelines for primary care providers on when to refer patients to the specialty pain clinic for management of opioid treatment) ($n = 1$).

Gaps in Support Processes for Opioid Prescribing

Although all administrators identified one or more supports for opioid prescribing, a few ($n = 2$) commented on the limitations or shortcomings of available supports. One administrator explained that although there were metrics and monitoring programs to support appropriate opioid prescribing, this information did not seem to be reaching the clinic providers:

> Uh, no. I have yet to see it—feedback [to prescribers]. I haven't seen the 360-communication loop. . . . Frankly, it all comes down to the prescriber as a single point of failure, looking at it [from] a systems point of view, and in my point of view, my opinion [is that it] is not a safe way. You want to have enabling infrastructure in place to help support that.

When asked about processes to support opioid prescribing, another administrator stated, "It starts and ends with me, for the most part. If I'm kind of on the fence about something, I would reach back to my colleagues that I trained with, if I was really struggling. But to me, it's pretty clear cut."

Challenges to Prescribing Opioids

We did not explicitly inquire during staff interviews ($n = 68$) about barriers or challenges specific to opioid and other medication treatment, but we did code these when they were mentioned, either while describing their approach to prescribing or when discussing barriers to high-quality care.[4] Although there were no opioid medication–related challenges that were endorsed by more than half of respondents, several themes emerged.

Inheriting Patients on Legacy Opioid Prescriptions

Some providers and administrators ($n = 15$) across all MTFs described the burden of taking over the care of patients who received opioid prescriptions from other MTF providers or from TRICARE network providers. As one provider explained, "Most of the time, what we're contending with [in terms of] patients on opioids is more of these legacy active-duty patients . . . and a civilian provider started them on Tramadol and now they're 400 mg Tramadol a day." Another clinician stated, "The patients I have picked up [from other providers], nobody does anything, it's just like, keep them on opioids." One respondent described their approach to this challenge, explaining,

> I apologize [to inherited patients on chronic opioids]. I'm like, "I'm sorry that someone put you on these [opioids]; this was the best guidance they had back then, they thought they were doing the right thing. But what we know now is that it is not helpful, and it can actually make your pain worse." And I really try to convince them to come off of it, knowing that it's going to be challenging.

Other Challenges to Prescribing Opioids

Furthermore, some staff ($n = 9$) across nearly all MTFs described prescribing barriers related to the EHR system and related metrics for opioid prescribing.[5] Respondents cited inadequate EHR supports for opioid prescribing, stating that they received plentiful pop-up messages about naloxone, but the EHR lacked features to direct providers to the right screen for co-prescribing of naloxone. Others discussed *alert fatigue* (i.e., feeling overwhelmed at the number of pop-up messages with warnings about opioid prescribing), or stated that the EHR frequently crashed and would be unavailable for long periods of time, thus impeding prescribing. There were also administrators who mentioned that opioid prescribing metrics were not easy to pull from the EHR, and several felt that the metrics themselves were not well designed (e.g., felt that naloxone was often suggested "even if it's exceedingly low clinical risk"). Several staff ($n = 5$) mentioned feeling overwhelmed or confused by the extent of oversight requirements for opioid prescribing (e.g., "I feel like the policies and procedures here were not very clear on what was expected . . . and then you ask around, and nobody else really knows").

---

[4] Elsewhere, we summarize staff-reported supports for the use of NPT (Chapter 6) and staff-reported overarching barriers to good pain care (Chapter 7).

[5] At the time of our interviews, MTFs were at different stages in the transition from AHLTA to the new EHR system, MHS GENESIS.

Nonopioid Medication Used for Chronic Pain

In this section, we summarize prescriber experiences providing nonopioid medication treatment. In a subsequent section in this chapter, we describe patient reports of medications received for pain in the past six months.

When asked, all prescribers ($n = 50$) endorsed providing nonopioid medication treatment to service members. It should be noted that we did not collect data about the conditions or indications for which the medications were used. The medications endorsed by the largest number of prescribers as being used most often to treat chronic pain were anticonvulsants (e.g., gabapentin) ($n = 42$), antidepressants (e.g., duloxetine and nortriptyline) ($n = 40$), and oral NSAIDs ($n = 39$) (Figure 5.2). Some prescribers mentioned frequently using non-NSAID topicals (e.g., topical capsaicin and lidocaine cream or patches) ($n = 22$), muscle relaxants (e.g., cyclobenzaprine) ($n = 20$), NSAID topicals (e.g., diclofenac gel) ($n = 16$), or acetaminophen ($n = 15$). Some ($n = 5$) endorsed frequent use of cannabinoids (e.g., Marinol). Several ($n = 4$) reported frequent use of oral dietary supplements, several ($n = 4$) endorsed frequent

FIGURE 5.2
Nonopioid Medications That Prescribers Reported Using Most Often to Treat Chronic Pain

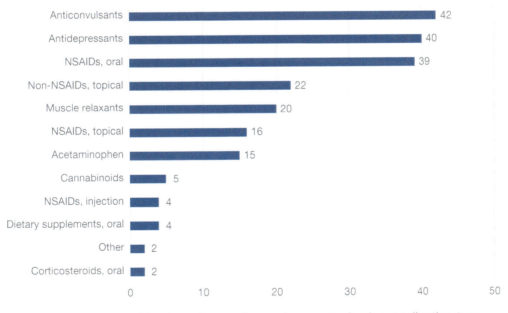

NOTE: Other includes ketamine and beta blockers. $N = 50$.

use of NSAID injection, and a few ($n = 2$) endorsed frequent use of oral corticosteroids. A few ($n = 2$) mentioned frequent use of other oral medications (e.g., ketamine and beta blockers).

Among frequent oral, topical, or injection NSAID prescribers ($n = 42$), many ($n = 21$) described using longer-acting oral formulations, such as meloxicam or celecoxib. As one provider explained, "I usually try to get [patients] onto a longer-lasting NSAID, such as Mobic [meloxicam] [or] naproxen, so that they remember to take it." Other prescribers reported frequent use of short-acting oral NSAIDs, such as ibuprofen. Some prescribers ($n = 16$) reported frequent use of topical formulations, such as diclofenac sodium 1 percent gel. As one provider stated, "I go for topical medications like diclofenac gel first. I really try not to use a lot of medications." A few prescribers ($n = 4$) reported frequent use of the injectable NSAID ketorolac to treat chronic pain.

Among the providers who prescribed anticonvulsants ($n = 42$), gabapentin and pregabalin were the most common, although there were also prescribers who mentioned using topiramate. A subset of these prescribers described using gabapentin or pregabalin specifically for neuropathic or nerve-related pain. One clinician stated, "[I would use] gabapentin if more nerve related, but if it's musculoskeletal, probably not." Another explained, "If fibromyalgia, I'll do pregabalin, or if neuropathic pain, I'll do gabapentin due to the evidence, but more recent clinical trials do not support it otherwise." Other providers reported using anticonvulsants without specifying the indication.

Among prescribers who reported commonly using antidepressants to treat chronic pain ($n = 40$), most ($n = 27$) mentioned duloxetine. The VA/DoD CPG cites weak evidence for its use in knee osteoarthritis and chronic low back pain (U.S. Department of Veterans Affairs and U.S. Department of Defense, 2022a; U.S. Department of Veterans Affairs and U.S. Department of Defense, 2020a), but we did not collect information about the specific pain conditions for which duloxetine was prescribed. Nonetheless, one provider shared, "Typically SNRIs [serotonin and norepinephrine reuptake inhibitors]—duloxetine—is the medication we most commonly use. It has good evidence for chronic musculoskeletal pain; it's been studied for that." Another stated, "Medication-wise, especially chronic pain, I've decided I'm a huge fan of Cymbalta [duloxetine]; especially if they have co-occurring depression." Other clinicians described using tricyclic antidepressants, such as amitriptyline and nortriptyline, remarking on the added benefit of such medications for co-occurring sleep issues or headaches. As one provider explained, "We do utilize tricyclic antidepressants for their pain benefit; they do help a lot of soldiers sleep a little better—we use amitriptyline and nortriptyline pretty regularly." The VA/DoD CPG notes that evidence is equivocal for the use of tricyclic antidepressants for low back pain (U.S. Department of Veterans Affairs and U.S. Department of Defense, 2022a).

Although invasive interventions were not the focus of this study, we report those that were cited by providers. Approximately one-quarter of prescribers ($n = 13$) reported frequent use of nonsurgical invasive medication and other treatments for chronic pain including injections of intra-articular or epidural corticosteroids ($n = 9$), intra-articular viscosupplementation ($n = 3$), trigger point ($n = 2$), and platelet-rich plasma ($n = 1$).

Medications Avoided or Used Less Often for Chronic Pain

There were several medications that some prescribers (n = 36) mentioned avoiding in their treatment of chronic pain. As mentioned earlier, over half of prescribers (n = 27) avoided opioids. Over one-quarter of prescribers (n = 14) stated that they try to minimize use of anticonvulsants, citing mixed evidence of efficacy or risk of causing drowsiness. The VA/DoD CPG notes equivocal evidence for the use of gabapentin or pregabalin for low back pain (U.S. Department of Veterans Affairs and U.S. Department of Defense, 2022a). As one prescriber explained, "Meds like gabapentin I will rarely use; the evidence is kind of mixed as to acute or chronic pain conditions that those [medications] help [treat]." Another stated, "I haven't used gabapentin recently because it can cause drowsiness, and with the airmen, you don't want that to happen . . . because if they got sleepy, they could not do their duty. And that's especially dangerous for those who carry a weapon." Some prescribers (n = 7) described minimizing or avoiding the use of antidepressants, citing doubts about their effectiveness. Others stated that they would instead refer patients to a BH provider. As one clinician explained, "I do not do psych drugs very often; I would generally get [patients] into counseling first." Another reported, "I don't personally [prescribe antidepressants]. At that point, we would send them to mental health for evaluation." A third clinician explained, "I'm not really sold on duloxetine; I haven't really had that great of an effect with it." Several respondents mentioned limiting use of NSAIDs (n = 4) because of provider or patient concerns about gastrotoxicity.

Medications Patients Received for Chronic Pain

We asked patients (n = 54) which medications, including opioids and nonopioids, they had received in the past six months for chronic pain. The majority (n = 45) reported having received an oral, topical, or injection medication (Figure 5.3). More than half of respondents mentioned taking oral NSAIDs (n = 30); the most common were ibuprofen (n = 21) and naproxen (n = 5). Approximately one-quarter of respondents mentioned taking muscle relaxants (n = 13). Some respondents reported taking anticonvulsants (n = 9); gabapentin was the most common (n = 6). Several respondents reported taking opioids (n = 4).

Some respondents reported taking antidepressants (n = 7); Cymbalta (duloxetine) was common (n = 4). Almost half of respondents taking antidepressants (n = 3) reported trying multiple antidepressants over the past six months; one respondent shared, "I have probably tried every single one; it's just not been helpful. Duloxetine [SNRI antidepressant], fluoxetine [selective serotonin reuptake inhibitor antidepressant], all the '-tines.' I've tried them [antidepressant medications] in the last few months." Although we asked patients to report on their medications for chronic pain, some patients reporting use of antidepressants might have received the prescription for a comorbid BH condition. Several respondents also mentioned taking acetaminophen (n = 5) or using topical NSAIDs (n = 4). A few respondents mentioned other topical preparations (n = 3) or sedatives (n = 3). A few patients mentioned receiving

FIGURE 5.3

Medications That Patients Reported Taking to Treat Their Chronic Pain

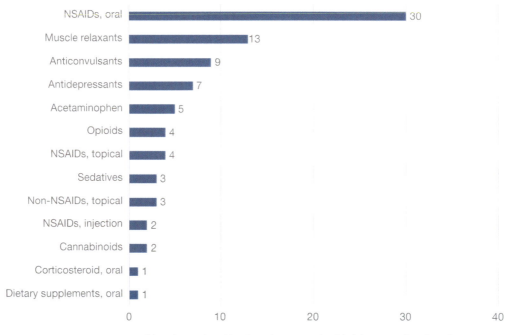

Number of patients who reported taking medication type

NOTE: Eight patients mentioned taking medication for chronic pain but did not recall the name or type of medication. $N = 54$.

NSAID injections ($n = 2$), and a few mentioned taking cannabinoids ($n = 2$). One patient reported taking oral corticosteroids, and one reported taking an oral dietary supplement.

More than one-quarter of respondents mentioned receiving one or more invasive medication treatment with injections ($n = 19$), including intra-articular or epidural corticosteroids ($n = 13$), trigger point ($n = 2$), nerve block ($n = 2$), and intra-articular viscosupplementation ($n = 1$). One respondent described the benefits and downsides of injections:

> So, the injections are always really beneficial—being the cortisone injections in my back. They can be almost a life-changer sometimes. The downside, and I know it's a negative, is you have to schedule the next one [each injection] in advance. I don't know if the previous one [injection] will be worn off or not [by the date of my next appointment]. I have to schedule three months in advance. If [pain relief from the previous injection] wore off, then I'm good and have [the next appointment] scheduled. If it didn't [wear off], I have to [reschedule for a later date]. Then they also do Botox for me on my back [at the pain management clinic], which is a new thing. It's been an amazing pain care technique, which I'[d] never had before.

Summary

In this chapter, we described themes from provider, administrator, and patient interviews with respect to the use or receipt of pharmacologic treatment for chronic pain. In keeping with the stepped-care approach, prescribers used nonopioid medication (along with NPT) for first-line treatment of chronic pain.

- **Opioid prescribing:** Most prescribers expressed trepidation about prescribing opioids for chronic pain, citing concerns about safety and addiction potential and the possible impact of opioid medication on service members' duties or military career. Prescriber confidence varied when it came to how or when to prescribe opioids for chronic pain and how to manage chronic pain patients already taking opioids that had been prescribed by another provider. Most prescribers minimized the use of opioids and expressed a preference for alternative pharmacologic and NPTs.
- **Programs to support appropriate opioid prescribing:** Administrators cited several programs to support providers in appropriate opioid prescribing at their MTFs. The most frequent support described was prescription monitoring feedback, followed by provider training and the availability of consultation with a pain clinic, pain champion, clinical pharmacist, or other specialist. Examples of challenges mentioned by prescribers related to pharmacologic treatment for chronic pain included managing patients whose opioid treatment had been initiated by another provider and frustration associated with EHR-based decision support, which could result in an excessive number of provider alerts and related provider alert fatigue.
- **Use of nonopioid medication:** Most prescribers reported that anticonvulsants, antidepressants, and oral NSAIDs were the most frequently used nonopioid medication for chronic pain. The next most frequently used medications were topical preparations (NSAID and non-NSAID), muscle relaxants, and acetaminophen.

CHAPTER 6

Nonpharmacologic Treatment for Chronic Pain

In this chapter, we describe themes from interviews with providers, administrators, and patients related to the use of NPT for chronic pain. NPT is a treatment choice for chronic pain used either alone or in conjunction with other treatments, including medication. Many different types of NPT exist, and several factors may affect which NPT is recommended by providers and accepted by patients. NPT is a key part of the stepped-care model for pain and, as noted in Chapter 4, it was cited as the preferred treatment for chronic pain among patient respondents. NPT provided in the MHS to service members with chronic pain may be associated with a reduced risk of long-term adverse outcomes (Meerwijk et al., 2020). Here we describe factors considered by providers in integrating NPT, administrator views on the extent to which NPT is utilized at their respective MTFs, and the types of NPT most used by providers to treat chronic pain. Additionally, we summarize feedback from providers and administrators on the biggest barriers to the use of NPT and themes from administrator interviews about the availability of organizational supports for integrating NPT.

Treatment Selection Considerations Specific to Nonpharmacologic Treatment

In this section, we describe factors considered by providers in the use of NPT, and the perspectives of administrators on the degree to which NPT is utilized at their respective MTFs.

Factors Considered by Providers in the Use of Nonpharmacologic Treatment

We asked providers ($n = 53$) about factors that influence whether they integrate NPT for service members with chronic pain. In follow-up probes, we prompted providers to consider the role of patient factors (e.g., patient presentation or preferences), structural or organizational factors (e.g., factors related to clinic operations, policies, or programs), and provider factors (e.g., provider preferences and perceptions of treatment effectiveness). Another follow-up probe prompted providers to consider which factors increase the likelihood that they would recommend NPT.

In responding to these questions, providers discussed both the *extent* to which they integrated NPT (i.e., near-universal use versus more-variable use) and the factors that influenced *which* NPT they integrated to treat service members with chronic pain. Overall, the most common considerations were patient preferences, treatment access or availability, and the type or severity of chronic pain condition.

Provider Use of Nonpharmacologic Treatment to Treat Service Members with Chronic Pain

Most providers ($n = 35$) across all MTFs told us that they use NPT with all or nearly all their chronic pain patients. They cited different reasons for this choice, such as the effectiveness of NPT, the lack of side effects of NPT—particularly relative to medication, or their belief in the superiority of NPT for service member populations (given their military duties). In contrast, some providers ($n = 18$) from across all MTFs described a more selective or variable approach to integrating NPT (i.e., not integrating NPT with all or nearly all their chronic pain patients). These providers discussed such factors as the limited availability of certain types of NPT or the importance of tailoring NPT to the patient's preferences or specific pain condition.

Patient-Related Factors

Regardless of whether they endorsed universal or selective use of NPT with their patients, nearly all providers ($n = 49$) across all MTFs cited patient preferences, willingness, or ability to engage in NPT as influencing their use of NPT to treat service members with chronic pain. As one provider summarized, "[I consider] their [patients'] time, their availability, and their willingness to proceed with whatever [nonpharmacologic] treatment I'm recommending." Another explained,

> In terms of psychotherapy [with an embedded BH consultant who is trained in cognitive behavioral therapy for chronic pain], honestly, I try to convince most of my patients that this is an intervention that they do want and that they could benefit from. I think we still have some barriers to what patients will understand about it and what they could potentially get out of it, but I will continue to try, because I've seen it make a huge difference in some of my patients and how they're able to experience their pain.

Additionally, most providers ($n = 31$) across all MTFs mentioned considering the type, severity, duration, or impact of the patient's pain condition, or the existence of co-occurring disorders, as a factor in determining whether or how to integrate NPT into their care. Said one provider, "I would say also [depending on] the length of their pain, like the chronicity, and if they've kinda failed the basics, then [we] definitely need to get them in to see [MTF psychologist] or . . . pain management." Another stated, "The more chronic it gets, the more I'm reaching deeper into the alternative treatments." Other providers mentioned the importance of assessing for comorbidities such as co-occurring BH conditions or obesity. Some providers (n = 19) across nearly all MTFs discussed the importance of assessing past treatments received, such as an experience of treatment failure or inadequate response with a previous trial of NPT. Some providers (n = 12) mentioned service member duties or responsibilities; most of these providers acknowledged that some service members' work or training schedules prohibited them from participating in NPT. Several providers (n = 4) discussed considering other patient-related factors, such as patient age, diet, or level of physical fitness.

Organizational Factors

The second most common factor mentioned by providers in describing their approach to the use of NPT was the availability of and access to NPT clinics or services, which was endorsed by most providers (n = 36) across all MTFs. In most cases, providers discussed limited NPT available within their clinic or MTF as a restricting factor in integrating NPT and described triage or referral methods for facilitating access for patients with the most severe pain to high demand services or referring eligible service members to other MTF facilities or programs with better access to NPT. As one provider explained,

> [Access is] the limiting step. I think a lot of our soldiers would want nonpharmacologic strategies if we had them available. The chiropractor, acupuncture, yoga—a lot more would want that. So, I would say that has a big influence on selecting, potentially—at a particular moment in time—a certain treatment.

Another provider from a different MTF stated, "A lot of patients would benefit, but I have to be very selective of who I send to my acupuncturist, psychologist, chiropractor. I would send everybody, but I can't. . . . So, I end up reserving it for [those patients] who would most benefit from it, who most want [the treatment]." In contrast, a smaller number of providers mentioned how robust access to certain services (e.g., physical therapy) shaped their decision-making around the use of NPT. Relatedly, some providers (n = 9) across nearly all MTFs cited the TRICARE reimbursement policy as a consideration in their use of NPT. Respondents reported that TRICARE does not reimburse for chiropractic care, acupuncture, or massage therapy if received through network providers, and many MTFs do not provide these services at their respective installations.

Fewer than one-quarter of providers (n = 6) also discussed challenges with appointment scheduling or wait times for NPT services, suggesting that the lack of appointment availability influenced their decision of whether to use NPT or which NPT to utilize. Other considerations made by providers included the availability of consultation with a pain clinic, pharmacist, or other provider to determine when or how to integrate NPT (n = 4), military policy related to medical treatment limitations prior to medical separation and disability determinations (e.g., patients under review by the Medical Evaluation Board not being eligible for certain MTF services or secondary gain of disability process motivating patients not to participate in NPT) (n = 3), and special MTF policies or programs (e.g., "Because of our unit and the multidisciplinary nature of our unit, a high percentage of patients who come through our clinic will have those ancillary [nonpharmacologic] treatments") (n = 3). One provider mentioned inadequate staffing for NPT as a factor, and another discussed administrative burdens and the challenge of not having enough time in the visit to integrate NPT (i.e., "I offer osteopathic manipulative therapy . . . but I don't have enough time to appropriately give that to our patients. . . . We could do dry needling as well . . . but the follow-up care would take too many time slots, which we can't really do.").

Provider Factors

Some providers (n = 20) discussed the role of their own preferences or beliefs about treatment as a factor in their decision of whether or how to use NPT to treat service members with chronic pain. The nature of these beliefs and preferences varied. Said one provider, "I think sometimes I would rather do the least invasive [treatment] for the most benefit to the patient. So, I would say, physical therapy is a great one. And I mean, really, the chiropractic is a good one." Said another provider,

> I prefer acupuncture, but I know not everybody is naturally inclined to have needles. So, I describe it to [patients]. . . . If they don't want it, I'm not upset or don't take offense to that, it just makes my day easier. Because it takes a while to do an acupuncture treatment. If I'm just doing a referral and sending them on their way, it takes less time. But I do it because it works and it's really helpful.

Relatedly, some providers (n = 17) discussed the perceived effectiveness of NPT as a consideration in their use to treat service members with chronic pain. Providers discussed NPT for which they felt the evidence base supporting treatment effectiveness was lacking (e.g., chiropractic care), whereas others discussed specific treatments that they perceived as being particularly effective (e.g., physical therapy). Additionally, some providers (n = 15) mentioned their clinical training or background as a consideration in which NPT to use, citing training or past experience in administering specific modalities, such as battlefield acupuncture or osteopathic manipulation.

Administrator Perspectives on the Degree to Which Nonpharmacologic Treatment Is Used

We also asked administrators (n = 15) about the degree to which providers at their MTF integrate NPT in their approach to managing chronic pain. Consistent with the feedback we received from providers, most administrators (n = 10) reported use of NPT with all or nearly all patients. Said one respondent, "I think [NPT is integrated] very highly. They [providers] do a very good job. That's been a big point of emphasis really over the last several years across the DoD and at this MTF as well, that's something we try to prioritize." Another administrator from a different MTF stated,

> That's our preferred method of treating patients—either acutely or chronically. As primary care providers, we are limited in what we can offer. And we know that even though we're

a small clinic, we're blessed with having the specialties in-house at least for pain purposes with the chiropractor and sports medicine. Especially since it's in-house, that's helpful.

A smaller number of administrators (n = 3) described selective or variable use of NPT, either because of limited availability and access barriers, inadequate TRICARE funding for certain NPT, or the variable scope of practice of available providers (e.g., "For example, for a while, we had people that were very much into auricular battlefield acupuncture as an adjunct. Those staff turned over, so it wasn't sustainably maintained."). A few administrators (n = 2) gave responses that made it difficult to determine the extent to which providers at the MTF integrated NPT into the treatment of service members with chronic pain, but they did emphasize efforts to reduce opioid use and provide treatment consistent with CPGs.

Nonpharmacologic Treatment Used or Avoided for Chronic Pain

In this section, we summarize perspectives of providers regarding the NPT used most often or avoided for the treatment of service members with chronic pain.

Nonpharmacologic Treatment Used Most Often

We asked providers (n = 53) whether there were types of NPT that they relied on most heavily, and if so, why. All providers (n = 53) endorsed one or more NPT that they used frequently.[1] In this section, we summarize overall trends in NPT used most often. We also provide a more in-depth review of provider comments regarding the most commonly used NPT. Figure 6.1 provides an overview of NPT that providers reported integrating most frequently to treat chronic pain.

Physical therapy was described by nearly all providers (n = 49) from all MTFs as an NPT they used often. The next most frequently cited NPT was BH care (e.g., referrals to a BH provider), which was endorsed by some providers (n = 23) across a majority of MTFs.[2] Other commonly mentioned NPT were chronic pain self-management (n = 19), chiropractic care (n = 17), and ice or cold therapy (n = 15)—all of which were endorsed by providers across all MTFs. Acupuncture was also cited by some providers (n = 18) across nearly all MTFs. Addi-

---

[1] Our codes did not distinguish between NPT administered by providers versus provided as a referral. Thus, in some cases, these NPTs were treatments the providers themselves were administering (e.g., a psychologist who primarily used psychotherapy for pain), whereas, in other cases, the NPTs were the referrals that the providers most frequently provided to patients (e.g., a primary care provider who primarily referred patients to the clinic psychologist for psychotherapy for their pain). Additionally, our codes did not distinguish between NPT that was available within the MTF versus that provided through a private-sector provider.

[2] BH care mentioned as part of treatment for chronic pain excludes care for comorbid BH conditions. Explicit mention of psychotherapy for pain was coded as its own category and is not included in BH.

FIGURE 6.1

Nonpharmacologic Treatment That Providers Reported Using Most Often to Treat Chronic Pain

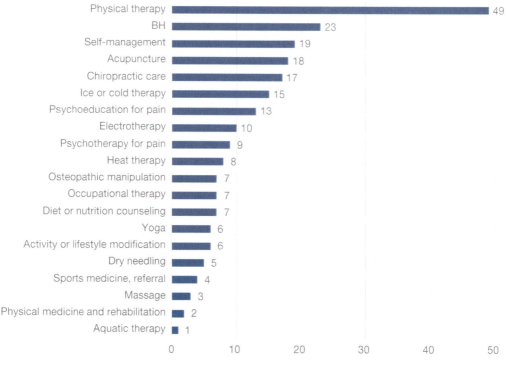

Number of providers who reported using each NPT type

NOTE: *N* = 53.

tionally, some providers (across all MTFs) reported frequent use of pain education and skills training (*n* = 13) and electrotherapy (*n* = 10), such as use of a transcutaneous electrical nerve stimulation (TENS) unit or other forms of electrical stimulation. Some providers, representing more than half of MTFs, reported frequent use of psychotherapy for pain (e.g., cognitive behavioral therapy for chronic pain) (*n* = 9), heat therapy (*n* = 8), and osteopathic manipulation (*n* = 7). Equal numbers of providers (across more than half of MTFs) mentioned occupational therapy (*n* = 7), diet or nutrition counseling (*n* = 7), yoga (*n* = 6), or activity or lifestyle modifications (*n* = 6) as their most used NPT for chronic pain. Several providers across more than half of MTFs (*n* = 5) reported frequent use of dry needling. Several providers reported frequent use of sports medicine referral (*n* = 4), massage (*n* = 3), physical medicine and rehabilitation (*n* = 2), or aquatic therapy (*n* = 1).

Physical Therapy

As discussed, nearly all providers (*n* = 49) across all MTFs reported frequent use of physical therapy. It was often described as a first-line treatment or as a first step in the treatment approach for chronic pain. Providers also appreciated the orientation of MTF physical therapy programs toward returning service members to a state of physical readiness for duty. Explained one provider of the physical therapy providers, "They only treat the active-duty population here, so they are very focused on everybody being physically ready. You know, return to full duty, or restricted appropriately. They don't treat any other beneficiaries. So, they're very active-duty-focused. Like, that's their mission." Other providers emphasized the ease of access to physical therapy. Some MTFs offered open access or *sick call* physical therapy, allowing service members to self-refer, and other MTFs had special physical therapy programs that were embedded in units or available only to a specific population, such as special forces.

In describing their approach to using physical therapy, numerous providers described using it in conjunction with self-management, nutrition counseling or weight management, or other activity modifications. As one provider stated, "Chronic pain is more individualized of an approach. Except activity modification, exercise prescription, and physical therapy, that's the mainstay of everything." Many providers we interviewed appreciated that physical therapy providers create specific rehabilitation plans for patients while also working on general flexibility and strengthening. Some providers described using resources in conjunction with a physical therapy referral, such as by providing handouts on recommended stretches or exercises for common musculoskeletal injuries or referring patients to similar materials on the Human Performance Resources website (Human Performance Resources, undated). None of the providers we interviewed described avoiding or minimizing the use of physical therapy.

Behavioral Health Care

As mentioned, some providers ($n = 23$) reported frequent use of BH care, such as a referral to a pain psychologist, an integrated BH consultant (i.e., a BH provider embedded in a primary care setting), or BH specialty care. References to BH care were much more common than specific mentions of psychotherapy for pain (such as cognitive behavioral therapy for pain), which were mentioned by only some of the providers. At some clinics or MTFs, a referral to BH care was a standard practice for most patients being treated for chronic pain (e.g., "I always offer it") or for any patients referred to a pain clinic (e.g., "If I am going to send somebody for TelePain services, I should send them to Dr. [pain psychologist]."). Other respondents described their use of BH care as being limited to chronic pain patients meeting certain conditions, such as those with co-occurring depression or sleep problems. Only one provider reported avoiding or minimizing the use of BH care for service members with chronic pain.

Self-Management

Of the providers who reported frequently using self-management strategies to treat service members with chronic pain ($n = 19$), most spoke of assigning home exercises or stretching. As discussed, these recommendations were often made alongside a referral to physical therapy. For providers at MTFs where physical therapy was readily available, the use of self-management exercises was a supplement to physical therapy. At MTFs where physical therapy was not as readily available, self-management strategies were described as a method to effectively use wait times until starting physical therapy. As one provider stated,

> The schedules for physical therapy patients are a bit harder; the system is not perfect for referrals, and it takes a bit longer for things to go through. We try to give patients their own means of starting things at home while they're waiting for the official referral to start, so we don't lose any time there.

None of the providers we interviewed described avoiding or minimizing the use of chronic pain self-management.

Nonpharmacologic Treatment Avoided or Used Less Often for Chronic Pain

We also asked providers ($n = 53$) whether there were types of NPT that they avoided or used less frequently in the treatment of service members with chronic pain, and if so, why. Most providers ($n = 37$) did not mention any NPT that they avoided. However, just over one-quarter of providers ($n = 18$) across all MTFs cited one or more types of NPT that they avoided or used less often.

Some providers ($n = 10$) mentioned avoiding or minimizing their use of chiropractic care, typically citing its limited availability or explaining that TRICARE does not reimburse for chiropractic care received through private-sector providers. Some providers ($n = 8$) mentioned avoiding acupuncture, often for similar reasons (i.e., limited availability and reimbursement issues). A few providers mentioned avoiding or less frequently utilizing other NPT, such as aquatics or water therapy ($n = 3$), psychotherapy for pain ($n = 3$), yoga ($n = 3$), psychoeducation for pain ($n = 2$), electrotherapy ($n = 2$), Tai chi ($n = 2$), osteopathic manipulation ($n = 1$), BH care ($n = 1$), or massage ($n = 1$).

Staff-Reported Barriers to Nonpharmacologic Treatment

We asked all staff ($n = 68$) what they saw as the biggest barrier to incorporating NPT in the treatment of pain for service members. There were no required follow-up probes. We coded for barriers and challenges to providing or overseeing NPT for the treatment of chronic pain that staff ($n = 68$) mentioned while answering other interview questions, such as our question about what gets in the way of delivering evidence-based treatment for pain (see Chapter 7). In this section, we summarize the overall themes with respect to barriers and challenges to NPT.[3] Although we did not probe for specific patient, provider or treatment, and organiza-

---

[3] Elsewhere, we summarize staff-reported barriers to medication treatment (Chapter 5) and staff-reported overarching barriers to good pain care (Chapter 7).

tional barriers to NPT, we coded and summarized themes in that format. Where applicable, we also indicate the NPT barriers that were the biggest barriers to providing or overseeing NPT for chronic pain.

All staff ($n = 68$) mentioned one or more barriers to NPT at some point during their respective interviews. Figure 6.2 provides an overview of the most common staff-reported barriers to incorporating NPT. These included organizational or structural barriers, which were mentioned by nearly all staff ($n = 64$), and patient barriers, which were mentioned by most staff ($n = 48$). One-quarter of staff ($n = 17$) discussed provider- or treatment-related barriers to NPT. We provide additional detail on these barriers in later sections.

Organizational Barriers

Organizational and structural barriers to NPT were the most common NPT-related barriers mentioned by staff across all MTFs, with most remarks centering on factors affecting patient access to care. Most staff ($n = 57$) across all MTFs cited barriers related to the lack of availability of one or more NPTs for active-duty service members, and over half of all staff ($n = 43$) across all MTFs cited these access barriers as the *biggest* barrier to integrating NPT. Said one provider in response to our question about the biggest barrier to integrating

FIGURE 6.2

Barriers to Incorporating Nonpharmacologic Treatment Most Frequently Cited by Staff

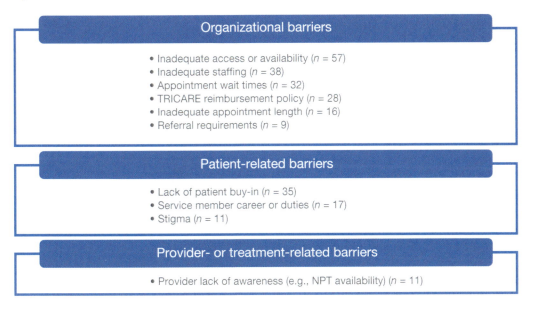

NOTE: The figure includes barriers to incorporating NPT discussed by 15 percent or more staff members. Administrator-reported barriers specific to appropriate opioid prescribing and staff-reported general or overarching barriers to pain care are excluded from this figure; they are discussed in Chapter 5 and Chapter 7, respectively. $N = 68$.

NPT, "Access. Actually, having the service and/or access to it. Availability." Most respondents spoke generally about limited access to NPT, although a subset of staff did mention specific treatments, such as physical therapy, acupuncture, or chiropractic care. Another NPT barrier that was frequently reported was scheduling delays or long wait times for NPT services, which was reported by nearly half of all staff (n = 32) across all MTFs. As one respondent explained, "Well, the barrier is probably the access. Because I know everybody wants to send their people for physical therapy and acupuncture. Sometimes it takes time, it takes a while." Another staff member stated,

> Everybody's fighting for that physical therapy. The physical therapy clinic here in [the MTF] has the first right of refusal to see a patient. So sometimes they'll resist sending somebody off-post for physical therapy [even when there is high demand or when staffing is inadequate]. So, it just means they [patients] may only be able to be seen in physical therapy once every two weeks [rather than more frequently], so that is frustrating for the patient, frustrating for us. Especially with COVID.

Another respondent described the implications of access and wait time barriers, remarking,

> I think some patients, if they can't get in, sometimes they get lost in the follow-up, so they just won't go. Then they don't get that care and they end up returning six to 12 months later, and the pain is still there. And we'll say, "Did you get in for physical therapy?" And they say, "No, I couldn't get in for three months," and then here we go again [push it out another few months].

Another structural NPT barrier that was commonly reported by individuals citing access and wait time issues was that of inadequate staffing, which was mentioned by over half of all respondents (n = 38) across nearly all MTFs. There was great variation in the type of staff discussed, but most respondents described challenges hiring and retaining staff for NPT, and some said that there were not enough billets for NPT providers at their clinic or MTF. As one respondent explained, "I think the access issue, as far as consistency and frequency of appointments—I think it's a personnel issue." Another respondent explained how these staffing barriers are particularly pronounced in primary care settings:

> At a large facility that has a carve-out for people who are specialists in pain, they have not just providers but [they] also have support staff that can manage a portfolio or population of patients that fit into that inclusion category. We are a primary care clinic, so chronic pain, while important, is on a list of other things that are important. So, you always get into these discussions of, do you make the capability, or do you buy the capability? And unfortunately, the resources we have in these four walls are the resources we get. We don't have a lot of slack in the system—a couple notable exceptions being the clinical pharmacist and embedded behavioral health specialist, as being key enablers of chronic pain management.

> We largely depend on the PCM to have training, awareness of resources beyond the four
> walls of the clinic, so we have to make that or grow that [capability].

Other respondents described the challenge of keeping staff members informed of available NPT resources or the difficulty of training up clinic providers on interventions, such as battlefield acupuncture, in light of high rates of turnover. Another access barrier was that of the TRICARE reimbursement policy, which was discussed by some staff (*n* = 28) across all MTFs. Numerous respondents stated that TRICARE no longer reimburses for TENS units, and respondents stated that TRICARE does not pay for acupuncture, yoga, chiropractic care, or massage unless these services are provided at the MTF. Said one respondent, "I can send somebody to a chiropractor [at the MTF], but it may be four months before they get their first appointment because there [are] two of them. So, it's, 'Sure, go for it, but you'll probably have to pay out of pocket in town, because TRICARE doesn't cover it.' Same thing in acupuncture." Finally, with respect to access to NPT clinics, some staff (*n* = 16) across most MTFs mentioned that the short length of appointment visit time was a barrier to integrating NPT, particularly in primary care settings. Said one provider,

> One [barrier] I would say is time at the primary care level. Because a lot of that is patient
> education and establishing that relationship and rapport with your patient for education
> about pain. And it can sometimes be very difficult to do that in a 20-minute or 15-minute
> appointment. . . . And then the other [barrier], again, it's just patient expectation. And the
> fact that they maybe are expecting when they come in to just have an easy answer, which is
> maybe the pharmacologic treatment, as opposed to the other components of it, which are
> much more time and effort intensive. So, [I] think those are the two big drivers.

Other staff made similar remarks (e.g., "Sometimes [I manage to get] only few details in a visit, and . . . when [patients] come to a medical provider . . . some are not ready to admit that [they are in pain], so it takes time to crack open what they're exercising [or how they are managing their pain].").

Additionally, some respondents (*n* = 9) mentioned referral barriers, such as requiring all chronic pain patients to receive a certain NPT before being seen in pain management, despite adequate availability of that service. Other staff members (*n* = 6) discussed NPT barriers related to Medical Evaluation Board review and associated disability-related assessments (e.g., "I think the other burden is the secondary gain of that VA [disability] rating because half of the patients just want to document they have back pain so when they get out [it's already been documented]."). Several staff (*n* = 4) mentioned care coordination barriers to NPT (e.g., "there are a lot of missed appointments. Some say it's just confusion and depending on if they have case management or multiple specialties involved. . . . So there is a smorgasbord of mixed treatments and expectations . . . there is a lot of delay."). Others (*n* = 4) remarked on limited resources associated with their MTF size (e.g., "I definitely think resources in this area [are a barrier]. I've been at bases that have had more-comprehensive pain places. We're a small clinic."). A few respondents (*n* = 3) discussed MTF or DHA program or policy barriers to NPT (e.g., lack of focus by the MTF or DHA on chronic pain prevention). One mentioned EHR-related barriers to NPT. Last, a few staff ($n = 3$) mentioned other structural barriers to NPT, with one perceiving a "failure of leadership" to provide adequate support for intensive NPT programs.

Patient-Related Barriers

Patient-related barriers to NPT were also commonly reported by staff. More than half of staff ($n = 35$) across all MTFs reported challenges related to patient lack of buy-in or interest in NPT. Said one provider, "There are some patients that are not receptive to nonpharmacologic [treatments]. So I think that can be a barrier, although we don't see that very often." Another respondent stated,

> I would say the biggest would be patient expectations. They expect to—I think we're in an instant gratification–type world—I want to take a pill and it will be gone by tomorrow. And whenever you do something like physical therapy it's going to take six to eight weeks to improve; patients don't like that, so they're not as receptive to it. They want something [that will work] right now.

Some staff ($n = 17$) cited service member duties as a barrier to use of NPT, explaining that service members' schedules prohibited them from attending NPT appointments or that frequent deployment and permanent-change-of-station cycles make medication a more viable treatment option. Additionally, some staff ($n = 11$) discussed stigma as a barrier to the integration of NPT, particularly BH treatment (e.g., "There is some concern. Like, if you refer somebody to the IBHC [integrated behavioral health consultant], they say, 'I don't have a mental problem.' So, getting past that to understand it's more—it's [about] more of a holistic approach to treating pain."). Several respondents ($n = 4$) discussed barriers related to the pain condition or prognosis (e.g., patients tending to seek medical help later in the course of their chronic pain because of fear of implications to the service member's career). Several staff ($n = 4$) mentioned unit or command barriers to NPT (e.g., lack of support for service members' time away from duties for appointments), and a few staff ($n = 3$) mentioned other patient-related barriers to NPT (e.g., past negative experiences with NPT that shaped future willingness to engage in treatment).

Provider- or Treatment-Related Barriers

One-quarter of staff ($n = 17$) across nearly all MTFs discussed provider- or treatment-related barriers to NPT. The most common was a lack of provider awareness about available nonpharmacologic services, which was cited by some staff across nearly all MTFs ($n = 11$).

Other Barriers

Some staff (*n* = 7) across most MTFs mentioned other barriers to the integration of NPT in treating service members with chronic pain, such as the COVID-19 pandemic. Said one provider, "I have to be honest with you, because it's not only this facility; sometimes it has been chaotic during the pandemic." A provider at a different MTF explained, "Especially, you know, with the pandemic, short staffing . . . we do have to send out to off-base [treatment]. And sometimes we just depend on the local medicine system to support it."

Processes to Support Providers in Integrating Nonpharmacological Treatment

We asked administrators (*n* = 15) whether there were any processes in place to support providers in using NPT, such as provider education, ongoing monitoring, or feedback.[4] Apart from these examples, there were no consistent probes. Despite this, we coded and analyzed NPT supports in a structure similar to other interview questions, categorized by organizational, provider, and patient factors.

All administrators (*n* = 15) cited one or more supports for the integration of NPT in their replies. All administrators (*n* = 15) across all MTFs mentioned organizational or structural facilitators, and most (*n* = 11) across nearly all MTFs described provider supports. We provide additional detail in later sections.

Organizational Supports

Although limited access was identified as a barrier to integrating NPT, with respect to organizational supports, over half of all administrators (*n* = 8) across most MTFs cited adequate availability of one or more NPT services. As one respondent explained, "So, we are unique in that we do have acupuncture here. A lot of MTFs don't. We also have a chiropractor here and a lot of MTFs don't." Another administrator stated, "We have an in-house physical therapist who has been great having walk-in hours, has pretty good availability. So, it's been great having him to help provide that care in our clinic." Walk-in or on-call services were often a feature of the NPT that administrators cited as being assets, including for the treatment of chronic pain (i.e., in addition to acute pain). As another respondent explained, "We have physical therapy that is very approachable and very good if we want to get somebody in with them. We maintain sick call, so that patients can come in in the morning if they have a pain thing going on."

Additionally, over half of administrators (*n* = 8) across nearly all MTFs mentioned the availability of consultation with a pain champion, pain medicine physician, or other special-

---

[4] Elsewhere, we summarize administrator-reported supports for appropriate opioid prescribing (Chapter 5) and staff-reported overarching facilitators of good pain care (Chapter 7).

ist to support the use of NPT. Most of these respondents described consultation occurring during clinic- or hospital-wide meetings, quarterly peer review sessions, or Project ECHO conferences. Others described a general environment in which providers could freely consult with one another to discuss the use of NPT for chronic pain. Lastly, some administrators ($n = 5$) across some MTFs (all of which had pain clinics) discussed MTF or DHA policies to support NPT, such as the allocation of protected funding to interdisciplinary pain management centers (IPMCs) to support the provision of additional services (e.g., "the DHA mandates that got me my social worker and psychologist"). Fewer respondents described care coordination supports ($n = 3$), other organizational supports (e.g., tracking systems for "high utilizers") ($n = 3$), helpful referral practices ($n = 2$), or staffing supports ($n = 1$).

Provider Supports

Of the provider supports that were mentioned by administrators, provider post-professional training was the most common: It was endorsed by most administrators ($n = 10$) across nearly all MTFs. Some of these trainings were led by pain care champions or by a specialty pain medicine physician who reviewed pain care best practices, available treatment resources, or relevant policies. As one pain clinic administrator explained, "We try to educate the other clinics and other clinicians as to what we do here and what we can provide [at professional] staff meetings and things that we have, like, hospital-wide meetings." There was also some overlap with mentions of Project ECHO or trainings delivered during all-staff meetings. Another administrator from a pain clinic stated, "We have ECHO conferences that [a pain medicine physician] helps arrange, so that we can interface with primary care providers outside of this clinic or outside of this hospital who want input on complex cases." Other respondents discussed trainings that were available to providers on specific NPTs (e.g., battlefield acupuncture) or trainings attended as annual symposia or continuing medical education (CME). Of note, all but one of the administrators who mentioned training supports were from MTFs that have pain clinics; administrators from MTFs with no pain clinic were less likely to mention provider post-professional training to support NPT. Additionally, a few administrators ($n = 2$) mentioned the stepped-care model that encouraged NPT use.

Patient Perspectives of Nonpharmacologic Treatment

We began our interviews with patients ($n = 54$) by asking about the types of treatment they had received for pain in the past six months. Nearly all patients ($n = 50$) across all seven MTFs reported that they received some form of NPT; physical therapy ($n = 36$) was reported as the most widely received NPT. Figure 6.3 provides an overview of NPT that patients reported receiving. The second most common NPT received was chiropractic care ($n = 20$); patients from all seven MTFs reported that they received chiropractic or manual adjustment and/or joint realignment. Other commonly reported NPTs were acupuncture ($n = 9$), followed by self-management (e.g., home exercises or stretching, braces or insoles, and body mechanics or

FIGURE 6.3

Nonpharmacologic Treatments That Patients Reported Receiving in the Previous Six Months

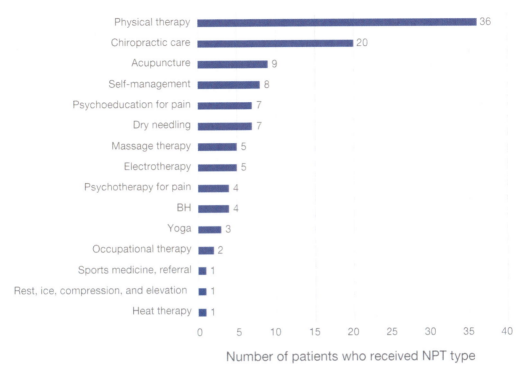

NOTE: N = 50.

ergonomics) (n = 8); psychoeducation for pain, including participation in a pain skills group or pain management class (n = 7); and dry needling (n = 7). NPTs that were less frequently received included massage therapy (n = 5), electrotherapy (n = 5), psychotherapy for pain (n = 4), BH (n = 4), and yoga (n = 3).

As noted, for the patients interviewed (n = 54), physical therapy was the most commonly mentioned NPT utilized (n = 36). Like providers, patients described physical therapy as the first line of treatment for their pain conditions—they were either referred by their PCM or self-referred. Patients noted that physical therapy included a variety of treatments, from stretching and strengthening exercises to icing and heating affected areas, and "advice on how to cope with [pain]." One patient commented on their experiences at physical therapy, explaining, "I'm trying to focus more on the strengthening and mobility, or ensuring my injury is not going to be affecting my daily life . . . making sure I'm strengthening that portion of my injured body . . . along with improving the mobilization of it." Another described their physical therapy routine as follows: "They heat [the affected pain area] when I first get there, and then I'll do different stretches and exercises, and then they'll . . . do ice at the end. That's helping with the pain."

However, patient reactions to physical therapy were mixed: Although certain patients spoke highly of it and said that they benefited greatly from physical therapy, others mentioned that they saw little to no improvement with physical therapy or felt additional pain after, which ultimately led to them halting treatment. As one patient described, "I think the end of my physical therapy was pretty close to six months ago, when I quit going to that because I wasn't getting any production out of it, any improvements, I mean [from physical therapy]." Another patient who had a similar experience said, "From my perspective, if you're progressing or not progressing or declining, they continue to just give physical therapy rather than doing more."

Additionally, patients mentioned the benefit of having physical therapy embedded in their units. For example, a patient stated, "I've got a physical therapist that sits on my squadron, so I go talk to him multiple times per week. And it's like, 'How is this feeling, let's try this or that.' I'm fortunate we have the SOCOM [Special Operations Command] things in our squadron to help. Not everyone can walk in and see a physical therapist three days per week." Others also spoke highly of their specific treatment embedded in their special forces units, including a suite with their own billeted providers, two to three physical therapy providers, and relatively easy access to the treatment and facility.

Patients also described other NPT utilized in conjunction with their physical therapy, including pain management classes, chiropractic care, acupuncture, and dry needling. For example, multiple patients mentioned receiving back adjustments from their physical therapy provider. One patient mentioned, "When I finally got in to see the physical therapy for specific—for [my] back—he did an adjustment, like on the table, where he stretched me out a little bit and tried to unlock my problem area." Another stated, "Then with her [physical therapist] being the chiropractor, she just like helped me and adjusted my back as I needed it." Patients also mentioned that if they saw no improvement with physical therapy, they were referred to chiropractic care next: "I did physical therapy and nothing worked; they said we'll try something else, and that's when they sent me to the chiropractor."

Summary

In this chapter, we described themes from interviews with providers, administrators, and patients related to the use of NPT for chronic pain.

- **Use of NPT:** Overall, most providers and administrators reported universal use of NPT with chronic pain patients. Nearly all providers cited patient preferences or willingness to engage in treatment as factors most often considered in using NPT. Most providers cited availability of NPT, and over half mentioned the type, severity, duration, or impact of the patient's pain as key considerations. Physical therapy was by far the most common NPT cited as being used most often by providers. After physical therapy, the most commonly used NPTs according to providers included BH care, chronic pain self-management, acupuncture, and chiropractic care. Most patients reported having received physical therapy in the six months prior to the interview, and some reported receiving chiropractic care. Fewer cited having received acupuncture or self-care management.

- **Barriers to the use of NPT:** Despite the popularity of NPT across all MTFs, over three-quarters of staff reported limited availability of NPT as the biggest barrier to integrating NPT into pain care. Approximately half of all staff also cited inadequate staffing, long appointment wait times, reimbursement issues related to NPT provided in private-sector care, or a lack of patient buy-in as barriers to the use of NPT. Other providers noted that constraints on patients' time and military duties may act as barriers to their using NPT.

CHAPTER 7

Facilitators and Barriers to High-Quality Pain Care

In this chapter, we describe themes from interviews with staff (administrators and providers) and patients on facilitators and barriers to the delivery of high-quality pain for service members. First, we describe staff perspectives on facilitators and patient perspectives on what aspects of their pain care went particularly well (referred to as *strengths*). We also review the barriers to high-quality pain care as reported by staff and patients.

Facilitators and Strengths

We asked staff to identify supports or facilitators that were helpful to them in the delivery of evidence-based pain care. Patients were asked to identify aspects of care that they felt had gone particularly well. We summarize the responses of both staff and patients. In each category, the results are presented from the most to least endorsed.[1] Figure 7.1 provides an overview of the most prominent facilitators and strengths.

Staff-Reported Facilitators

Staff (*n* = 68) were asked about their perceptions of what helped or supported them in delivering or overseeing high-quality pain care. Follow-up probes prompted staff to consider structural or organizational supports (e.g., clinic operations, policies, or programs) and provider supports (e.g., training or experience with treatment options). Elsewhere, we summarize staff supports specific to appropriate opioid prescribing (Chapter 5) and provider use of NPT (Chapter 6). The focus of this section is on more-general or overarching facilitators for high-quality pain care.

---

[1] Facilitators or strengths that are thematically similar are grouped into one report heading or category. The facilitator or strength in each category that was endorsed by the largest number of respondents is what determines the overall order of that category in the report.

FIGURE 7.1

Facilitators Most Frequently Endorsed by Staff and Strengths Most Frequently Endorsed by Patients

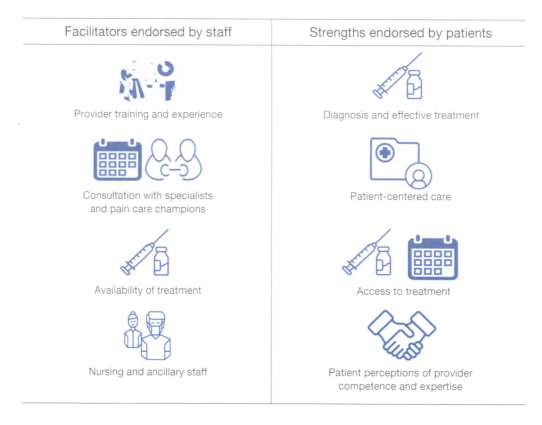

Facilitators endorsed by staff	Strengths endorsed by patients
Provider training and experience	Diagnosis and effective treatment
Consultation with specialists and pain care champions	Patient-centered care
Availability of treatment	Access to treatment
Nursing and ancillary staff	Patient perceptions of provider competence and expertise

NOTE: The figure includes facilitators endorsed by 15 percent or more staff members (N = 68) and strengths endorsed by 15 percent or more patients (N = 54). Staff facilitators specific to appropriate opioid prescribing and provider use of NPT are excluded from this figure, as they are discussed in Chapters 5 and 6, respectively.

Provider Training and Experience

Most staff (n = 30; administrators = 5, providers = 25) discussed ongoing provider training in pain care as a key facilitator. Administrators highlighted a breadth of training opportunities, including continuing medical education focused on pain care for primary care providers, weekly Project ECHO sessions, and training sessions led by pain champions. Providers also highlighted similar training opportunities, with Project ECHO sessions being the most commonly mentioned. One provider described the utility and future direction of such learning opportunities:

> We do a provider off-site twice a year, just lectures, and we get CME for it. And we usually have people from other specialties. But I think that would be a really good opportunity for someone from the pain clinic to come in and give us suggestions on what we need to do before we send someone [to the pain clinic], or anything like that. Just because from my

own personal experience, I don't think I was taught a whole lot about chronic pain management, but that is something that we could all benefit from.

Provider formal education and other prior experience (i.e., training received prior to their current role) were also identified by staff (n = 21; administrators = 0, providers = 21) as key facilitators to delivering good pain care. Half of these providers discussed the role of their medical school or residency training, whereas others mentioned other types of relevant experience (e.g., nursing school, military service, and serving as a pain champion). Providers who highlighted their prior experience as helpful discussed collaborating across specialties to address pain and having years of experience in pain management. A provider summarized, "my training and practice and having [sports medicine] patients and the experience of practicing with those patients and seeing those patients has developed my skill set [for treating pain] more."

Consultation with Specialists and Pain Care Champions

Almost half of staff (n = 29; administrators = 7, providers = 22) discussed consulting pain care specialists and other providers as a key facilitator of providing effective pain care. For example, one provider stated, "being able to work with the pain clinic [and] different colleagues I've worked with on the way . . . all of these things I've picked up along the way I think have contributed to success." Another provider and pain champion remarked,

> Whenever I first got started here as the pain champion, our head of the pain management department, they came over . . . they actually showed up in the clinic face-to-face to help with any patients we weren't quite sure with, [and] they were always available if we needed to call and ask, "Hey, do you think this treatment is available?" So just the resource in pain management specialty and the relationship that we have has been awesome.

Relatedly, staff (n = 16; administrators = 9, providers = 7) highlighted the role of pain care champions as a support. As one staff member shared, "They're kind of the central command point of contact for sources of higher-level policy environments, as well as coordination for training." Similarly, some staff (n = 11; administrators = 3, providers = 8) noted the role of clinical pharmacists in supporting health care decisionmaking.

Availability of Treatment

The availability of certain pain care treatments was also mentioned by some staff (n = 14; administrators = 2, providers = 12) as a facilitator to delivering high-quality pain care. In some cases, staff discussed the advantages of having a pain clinic or treatment program at the MTF. For example, one administrator stated, "We have a robust pain management program and fellowship here, and I think that's great. I think the Navy has invested heavily in subspecialties that deal with acute and chronic pain." Other staff made general comments about their clinic's ability to meet patient needs for care. Providers overwhelmingly highlighted the importance of the availability of a pain management clinic or other specialty services (e.g., orthopedics); many emphasized the benefit of their being located in the same facility or nearby. A provider stated, "Here, with pain management in-house, it is nice to be able to refer patients in-house. Just so that they are not having to wait to be seen off-base." One provider emphasized the benefits of having access to ancillary services, such as X-ray and MRI on-site to support pain care. Providers also mentioned the ability to refer certain patients to special clinics or programs for receipt of multiple services, such as to special clinics for patients with a history of traumatic brain injury.

Nursing and Ancillary Staff

Other staff ($n = 11$; administrators $= 2$, providers $= 9$) referenced nursing and ancillary staff across various positions at their MTFs, in some cases emphasizing the importance of such staff—particularly nurses—in coordinating care. Said one provider, "What has helped is having good nursing staff. I think my pain patients, they like to know who the nurse is that they can call if they have a flare-up so they can let me know what's going on." Another provider remarked, "Nurse case managers are super helpful . . . [they] will know what in the area we can do, or if I need to facilitate getting [patients] to another MTF for services we may need there."

Other Facilitators

Other facilitators endorsed by staff members are described here.[2]

Strategies for Extending Length of Visits

Some staff ($n = 8$; administrators $= 3$, providers $= 5$) described the ability to extend pain care visits for existing patients through flexible scheduling as a facilitator. Primary care visits are typically limited to about 20 minutes, which could limit a provider's ability to adequately assess and manage patients with complex needs (Kottke, Brekke, and Solberg, 1993; Neprash et al., 2021; Yarnall et al., 2003). Administrators mentioned establishing informal guidelines allowing flexibility for longer appointments with complex pain patients when needed. Providers discussed advocating for additional time; one provider established their own method of double-booking appointments to ensure that 40 minutes could be allocated for patients with chronic pain.

Decision Support Tools

Staff ($n = 8$; administrators $= 4$, providers $= 4$) spoke of the advantages of EHRs and decision support systems. Administrators highlighted that the AHLTA EHR was helpful as long as the documentation was clear and longitudinal pain scores could be viewed.[3] One adminis-

---

[2] Facilitators discussed here were endorsed by fewer than 15 percent of staff members and were not thematically related to one of the aforementioned facilitators that *were* endorsed by at least 15 percent of staff members.

[3] At the time of our interviews, MTFs were at different stages in the transition from AHLTA to the new EHR system, MHS GENESIS.

trator discussed the Health Experts Online Portal (HELP) system, a virtual and protected consultative service to discuss complex patient cases. Another administrator offered how they felt existing referral guidance facilitated pain care delivery. Providers acknowledged the benefits of AHLTA templates, particularly for pain care assessment, and a centralized medical record with the ability to view patient records of pain care received at other MTFs. Another provider discussed the utility of algorithms or guidelines that support providers in making referral decisions.

Relatedly, staff ($n = 6$; administrators = 2, providers = 4) discussed facilitators specifically related to the use of CPGs or the stepped-care model for decision support. When asked about supports for the delivery of evidence-based care, one provider stated, "Clinical practice guidelines. I learned not too long ago, within the last couple of years, that we actually had one for pain. . . . So, using the CPGs and following some of those recommendations for pain control." Another provider explained, "There is a DHA stepped approach where it kind of outlines and breaks down different modalities you can use." An administrator similarly highlighted the role of the DHA stepped-care model, which they felt adequately described different treatment modalities for health care providers. Similarly, several staff ($n = 4$; administrators = 0, providers = 4) spoke of the utility of patient assessment tools in supporting the treatment of chronic pain. They all highlighted PASTOR, mentioning that it enables providers to track longitudinal patient self-reported outcome data and assists patients in understanding their progress while receiving pain care. One of these providers further emphasized the similar value of the DVPRS.

Care Coordination

Relatedly, staff ($n = 7$; administrators = 2, providers = 5) highlighted mechanisms to support care coordination and continuity of care. Providers echoed their remarks about the advantages of having nursing or ancillary staff to support care coordination. Said one provider, "If [the patient has] ever been given that ICD [International Classification of Diseases]-10 code 'chronic pain,' we do have a pain care coordinator nurse who helps triage those patients. And if they've ever seen [the MTF psychologist], she'll reach out to them to get in contact with them." Administrators emphasized Project ECHO meetings as opportunities for discussing complex cases, the role of practice managers, and the importance of open communication between providers.

Staff Commitment to Patients

Some staff ($n = 5$; administrators = 2, providers = 3) highlighted the perceived dedication and compassion of providers and other staff members. Said one provider, "I think our personnel and quality of people is the number one."

Unit- and Command-Related Facilitators

A few staff ($n = 3$; administrators = 1; providers = 2) discussed unit- and command-related facilitators. For example, one provider highlighted the important benefits of receiving support from commanders, stating, "the commanders, knowing me . . . and knowing that [I] am not going to try to take all [their] people out of their gear and take their guns at once, [is helpful]. So getting [commanders'] buy-in in how I am treating their members is helpful."

Patient-Reported Strengths

We asked patients (n = 54) what aspects of their pain care had gone particularly well. There were no specific follow-up probes.[4] Overall, nearly all patients (n = 50) endorsed one or more strengths, whereas several (n = 4) were unclear or did not identify any strengths. Common themes included diagnosis and effective treatment; patient-centered care; access to treatment and availability of appointments; provider competence and expertise; and other strengths, such as customer service and uncomplicated care navigation.

Diagnosis and Effective Treatment

The most common patient-reported strength or aspect of care that had gone well was patients receiving effective treatments (n = 22). Patients who endorsed this theme described feeling grateful that their condition had improved. For example, patients felt that such treatments as physical therapy, trigger point injections, chiropractic care, or treatment in a pain management clinic, helped them with their range of motion, mobility, and ability to perform daily activities. One patient remarked that after seeing the chiropractor, "[I felt a] boost in the right direction to help me invigorate outside the office and outside of medical treatments."

Relatedly, some patients (n = 11) emphasized that they appreciated having providers who took the time to carefully diagnose their pain condition and provide treatment options for their pain. One reported how a physical therapist determined that the patient had been misdiagnosed, and after performing the correct treatment adjustment, "I had very little pain compared to the amount of pain I was in when I got there. So, I actually appreciate his service. He's been the most effective person." A patient shared how a physical therapist performed a series of stretches for his shoulder, and the issue resolved. He stated, "I would say the physical therapy clinic has been a shining light in an overall dull situation of the medical care at [this MTF] so far." Another stated,

> I think honestly the past six months have been the best part because we know what the problem is. I've gone ten years without knowing that there is a problem with the hopes it will just get better. Now I actually know that there is something wrong.

Other patients observed how they felt their care improved once an MRI identified the root cause of their chronic pain. When asked what aspects of their care had gone well, one

---

[4]   Unlike with staff interviews, we asked patients about strengths at only one point in the interview (i.e., we did not ask patients to identify strengths specific to opioid prescribing or use of NPT). Thus, although we discussed staff facilitators in three separate chapters (facilitators of appropriate opioid prescribing in Chapter 5, facilitators of provider use of NPT in Chapter 6, and facilitators of good pain care in Chapter 7), patient strengths are discussed in this chapter only.

patient stated, "The progression after the MRI and going into the specialty care. . . . The way things actually started happening after that. I started getting the actual progress on things and moving forward with the treatments and possibilities."

Patient-Centered Care

The second most common theme from patients about what went well was having a provider who was understanding, communicated well, or supported patients in their choice of treatment (*n* = 20). Some patients endorsing this theme spoke highly of open lines of provider-patient communication and provider-provider communication. Patients felt that providers who were genuine and communicated directly were assets to their pain care treatment. Positive aspects of provider-to-patient communication included providers thoroughly explaining their approach to care, step by step. One stated, "[My provider] generally cares about my quality of life. She listens, we talk, and she never comes off and says 'This is what I'm going to give you.' She'll try to figure out what kind of lifestyle I live first." Provider efforts to educate patients about pain care were another aspect of communication that patients appreciated. Increasing the patient's knowledge about pain care included articulating various paths that patients could take for their pain treatment. A patient explained,

> It's different from 20 years ago to, "just take it and keep going," to now, where there has been a push to include to patients for what issue is, listen to what patient is going through, and trying to work from there, kind of like a team, in that sense.

Another patient described a physical therapist who was passionate about her job, remarking, "Because she was so passionate, she wanted to help me and teach me what was causing [the pain] so I could be more educated about the topic, too. I prefer that over prescriptions. . . . Because now [with the physical therapy] I know why [I experience pain]."

Other patients who appreciated their providers underscored the importance of their provider's patient-centered approach or the fact that they acknowledged patient preferences or gave them a choice of treatment. As one patient commented, "[The providers] are doing more than a surface look [at the pain]." One service member spoke of the benefit of tailoring care (e.g., physical therapy) to each individual service member because it's too often done in a group. He commented,

> And then [in] physical therapy, they're working well with me on a one-on-one case. . . . [On] one of the bases that I was at, they did group physical therapy, where there was like one technician with seven or eight soldiers or airmen and they gave everyone the same standard workout. And then other ones, it's just been cut and dry, like this is a workout plan that they give to everyone here at this facility.

Patients also spoke of how providers listened to them and tailored treatment to the patient and their pain concerns. One patient remarked,

I would say the treatment, or the personnel handling the physical therapy, have been very respectful [and] at the same time very knowledgeable about making sure that we are doing physical therapy the correct way. Some physical therapy in places or some medical treatment facilities sometimes give you a piece of paper and you go follow this little piece of paper and they are not with you throughout the entire time. However, here, they pretty much go step by step with you the entire time, so it feels like they're on journey with you in regards to getting better.

Another patient commented on the shared decisionmaking with providers, "In terms of going forward, figuring out the right course of action for me, [providers] seem to be receptive, 'Okay, how we get you there, what do you want to do.' It seems helpful. I haven't felt like I've been shut down, or [been told] 'Hey, here's your candy, go gnaw on it.'"

Access to Treatment

Some patients ($n = 11$) reported that they were appreciative of having access to certain treatments for chronic pain. For example, one patient described access to chiropractic care, remarking, "You do TDY [temporary duty orders] or deploy and need to pull out of the system. Even during COVID, the fact that [the chiropractic provider] and the clinic were able to keep me in the system is pretty amazing." Another patient commented, "Availability has gone well. There is a lot more availability of different types of treatment here than previous places. . . . I had never heard of pain management before I came here."

Relatedly, some patients ($n = 8$) reported that a short wait time to scheduled appointments was a strength. For example, patients cited quick access to primary care appointments. One stated,

Getting in as quickly as possible [has gone particularly well at this MTF]. Generally, every time I've gone in to make an appointment or be seen, I'm generally seen within a week of, you know, making contact with the clinic.

Similarly, patients endorsing this theme and seen in primary care described the quick referral process to specialists and ancillary services. One patient explained, "I've never had like a long delay to where I have to wait three months to start physical therapy. It's been rapid; that's the best word to use. I'm able to get in right away, and the availability is great." According to another patient, referral processes were quick, and appointments were well coordinated and scheduled.

Patient Perceptions of Provider Competence and Expertise

Patients ($n = 11$) also spoke of their perceptions of their providers' competence, background, experience, and training and how that positively affected their pain care. One patient commented,

I think that the vast amount of knowledge [providers] have [is a strength to my pain care]. I could ask them pretty much anything, and even if they don't have it, they're willing to go find [it]. I find that really interesting and great to know, because I have more confidence in coming back and being able to get taken care of.

Said another patient, "I really do enjoy my providers. They're really smart, so I'm appreciative of that." Another patient described a specific pain medicine provider whose expertise and background enabled them to provide excellent care:

> If she doesn't know something, she's like, "I am going to talk to my circle of other pain management docs; we'll find an answer, we'll try something." She's been carrying my care along, and I don't think it's her job to do that, but she's been the one that makes herself available. She's [out on medical leave] now, I think, but for the most part, she's like, "Let me order the MRI rather than going through them."

Other Strengths

Other strengths endorsed by patients are described here.[5]

Supportive Front Desk Staff

Patients (n = 7) also indicated that customer service provided at MTF clinics by support and front desk staff was an important and positive part of their pain care. One commented, "The team that is on the front desk—they are helpful, kind, courteous, compassionate. It's like the first two people you see when you get there, and they're always . . . cheerful and in a good mood to make you laugh. Like, to me, that's what starts out the best part of treatment there." Another detailed the personal interaction he had with the staff:

> When I have an appointment [at the MTF], I have to see the ladies [front desk staff] over there in the front. And that's the first good thing. They always [are] smiling, telling you a lot of stuff [that's] good. So they recognize you and they talk to you, not just as a patient. I have one who called me "Rico Suave"; I love that.

Relatedly, a patient mentioned care navigation support through referral management that facilitated his ability to get an appointment with a chiropractor. He explained,

> I guess what she was doing was calling every day to try and see if there [were] cancellations [with the chiropractor], so I didn't have to. It was a huge help and when she found it, she called me and she's like, "Hey, can you go in tomorrow at 13:00." [And I was like], "Yes, please, thank you," and I rolled right in. And that kind of got me into the schedule so then I've been consistent and reoccurring [in chiropractic care] ever since. That is a big plus for me. Initially it was like, oh gosh, two months [wait]. And this referral management lady really did a lot over the course of a couple of days.

---

[5] Strengths discussed here were endorsed by fewer than 15 percent of patients and were not thematically related to one of the aforementioned strengths that *were* endorsed by at least 15 percent of patients.

Other Treatment-Related Strengths

Lastly, several patients (*n* = 5) discussed other treatment-related aspects of pain care, such as patient education, communication between providers, and care continuity. One patient spoke of a messaging portal and how it was a convenient way to communicate with providers without making appointments. Another described good communication between providers as a strength: "Care is something [that] is going to happen anyway; I think communication between all parties [has] been key. And I think it has allowed us to move along from one treatment to the next seamlessly." Other patients described specific treatments that involved peer education and increasing their understanding of pain, such as group pain management classes, which were cited as beneficial. A patient spoke of the importance of peer support:

> When I was going through first phase [of pain treatment], before being able to go to this [pain management] class, I felt like I was alone. I felt like I was the only person who understood what back pain was. . . . I didn't know it was common, or something that happens, and that it's okay to not feel okay and actually seeing that people who outrank me in these classes, I'm able to relate to it. In class, I can sit and talk to an E-7 [i.e., a senior noncommissioned officer] and he's like relating [to me]. I go back to my unit, same rank, blah blah blah, they tell me you should never leave, but this class, it made me feel more like a person instead of a number in the Army. It made me feel validated in what I was experiencing. All the knowledge too . . . that's helped.

Additionally, another patient stated, "I'm educating myself not just on the next five years, but also [for] when I'm 55 to 75. It's literally because of the care provided within clinics like this—pain management."

Barriers

Staff and patients were asked to identify barriers to pain care. Specifically, staff were asked to identify barriers to the delivery of evidence-based pain care. Patients were asked whether there was anything that had gotten in the way of receiving pain treatment. We summarize the responses of both staff and patients. In each category, the results are presented from the most endorsed to the least.[6] Figure 7.2 provides an overview of common barriers from both the staff and patient perspectives.

Staff Perceptions of Barriers to Delivering Evidence-Based Care

We asked staff (*n* = 68) to reflect on what got in the way of their ability to deliver or oversee evidence-based care for acute and chronic pain. Follow-up probes prompted staff to consider

---

[6] Barriers that are thematically similar are grouped into one report heading or category. The barrier in each category that was cited by the largest number of respondents is what determines the overall order of that category in the report.

FIGURE 7.2

Barriers to Pain Care Cited Most Frequently by Staff and Patients

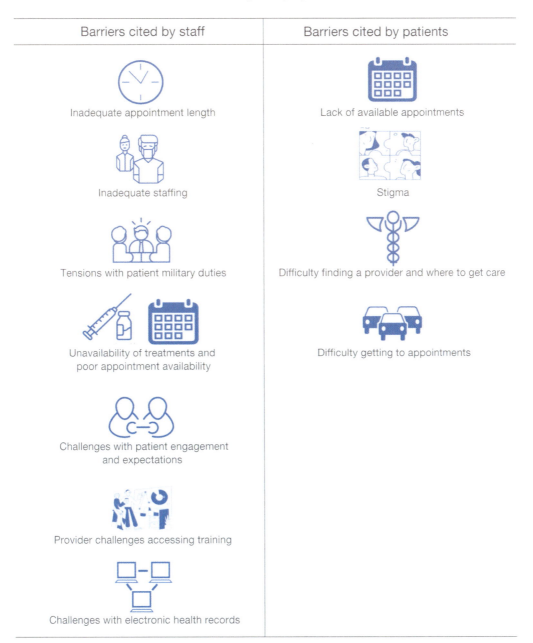

Barriers cited by staff	Barriers cited by patients
Inadequate appointment length	Lack of available appointments
Inadequate staffing	Stigma
Tensions with patient military duties	Difficulty finding a provider and where to get care
Unavailability of treatments and poor appointment availability	Difficulty getting to appointments
Challenges with patient engagement and expectations	
Provider challenges accessing training	
Challenges with electronic health records	

NOTE: The figure includes barriers discussed by 15 percent or more staff members (N = 68) and those discussed by 15 percent or more patients (N = 54). Staff barriers specific to appropriate opioid prescribing and provider use of NPT are excluded from this figure, as they are discussed in Chapters 5 and 6, respectively.

structural or organizational barriers (e.g., clinic operations, policies, or programs), provider supports (e.g., training or experience with treatment options), and service member barriers (e.g., duties, stigma, or financial barriers). Elsewhere, we summarized staff perspectives on barriers specific to medication treatment (Chapter 5) and use of NPT (Chapter 6). The focus of this section is on more-general or overarching barriers to high-quality pain care.

Inadequate Appointment Length

Limited time with patients was cited as a major barrier ($n = 25$; administrators = 6, providers = 19). Most of these administrators and providers highlighted how inadequate 15 to 20 minutes—the standard time allotted for a patient appointment—was to treat chronic pain. One administrator shared,

> Generally, the type of provider we have here is one that wants to care for the soldier and take whatever they say seriously. It is difficult when everything we see is in 20-minute appointment slots. In a primary care setting, it is hard to address most everybody's issues, if they have more than one [chronic pain issue], in a 20-minute session. Sometimes, that's the limiting factor.

Providers stated that having less time with patients limited their ability to provide education and obtain patient buy-in for treatment or commented on how lack of adequate time restricted their ability to cover aspects of the stepped-care model. One provider stated, "People just give people opiates because it's way easier than seeing them or weaning them off opiates. There is no time. No time in the MTF schedule. You cannot see chronic pain patients in less than 15 minutes, which is what the MHS expects you to do." Another provider explained,

> When we have to do education to the service member or to a patient about why we want to refer to behavioral health or include physical therapy, why not a quick fix, why we need their participation to be more active, it requires time. And that's how providers kind of get rushed into making some kind of decision about a treatment plan, which the patient may not agree with, if it didn't get explained properly.

One provider observed, "The pain patient needs more than 15 minutes. You know, I can remember a few years ago, we used to have what's called a pain clinic, and those patients had 30-minute appointments. . . . I know that's happening everywhere, but you know, they're not just cogs in the wheel. They don't all fit."

Separately, several staff ($n = 4$; administrators = 0, providers = 4) discussed the increasingly large or unmanageable size of their patient panel, with one stating that the DHA requires providers to see 20 patients per day (e.g., "DHA is hell bent on us seeing at least 20 patients per day. So patient load [is a barrier]"). Relatedly, two providers shared care continuity challenges that they described as stemming from not having enough time in the clinical day. They explained that care continuity becomes more challenging when the size of the patient panel increases, making it difficult to track a specific set of patients over time.

Inadequate Staffing

Staffing-related barriers ($n = 24$; administrators = 9, providers = 15) were one of the most common. Most respondents discussed being generally short-staffed, which negatively affected capacity to deliver primary care and specialty pain care services. A provider explained, "Just in the military world, we're underbudgeted, understaffed, and [facing] more budget cuts. It's really hard at an executive level to manage a full clinical repertoire with the inability of funding and resources." High staff turnover was also mentioned by some administrators ($n = 4$) and a provider. An administrator provided additional insight on this issue, indicating there is a lack of an active-duty pipeline of pain-specialty physicians. Relatedly, a provider stated that the mechanisms through which patients are reassigned to new providers in response to turnover can be ineffective and foster additional fragmentation and confusion. A provider also reflected on the challenges of having fewer billets:

> The Navy, in general, should look back to what the Air Force and Army have done . . . the Army, Navy, and Air Force decided to get rid of medical providers so that they could have more money in their pockets to do other things. Medicine was costing too much. Congress came back after COVID and said, "That's a bad idea." The Army and Air Force [had] made no changes [in staffing], but the Navy said, "It's too late, we've already closed those billets."

Staff ($n = 9$; administrators = 4, providers = 5) also shed light on challenges associated with the lack of nursing and ancillary staff across various positions at their MTFs. One provider discussed a nursing shortage, stating,

> We have zero nurses. So, we have people filling in from other areas of the hospital, which means we don't have that continuity of a nurse that really knows what's going on, our nurse manager. Where you don't have a consistent nurse manager, you don't deliver high-quality health care because there is no cohesion to the clinic.

Another reflected on the consequential impact of this, "If I had truly what I should have for support staff . . . I could probably see at least a third more patients in a day."

Tensions with Patient Military Duties

Some staff ($n = 23$; administrators = 5, providers = 18) described barriers related to the professional duties or careers of their service member patients. They acknowledged that professional demands could make it difficult to engage in treatment during regular office hours or at the recommended frequency. Others discussed how patients sometimes seemed reluctant to be forthcoming about the extent of their pain or its impact on functioning. Explained one provider,

> There is this phenomenon with my patients where they always have the service in the back of their mind, before they even consider booking an appointment with the doctor

> . . . sometimes I wonder if they're being fully forthcoming about the degree of their pain, that type of thing. I think it's kind of inherent to treating active-duty service members.

Other providers described how frequent permanent changes of duty station made it difficult to establish rapport or administer an extended course of treatment without interruption. One provider acknowledged how deployments could affect the course of treatment, stating, "So for people who get deployed, we tend to use pharmacological rather than nonpharmacologic [treatments], because obviously they are not around to do a nonpharmacologic thing."

Another related theme emerging from staff (n = 10; administrators = 4, providers = 6) was the notion that patients tended not to seek care early in the course of their pain condition for treatment. In this way, staff felt that patients allowed their pain to worsen in severity and chronicity before seeking care or referral services. One administrator shared,

> I notice when they are ready to retire. This has been hurting. . . . They are tough on them-selves. They put up with this pain and then they are ready to retire, and they come in with a whole load of problems, which we have to sort out so that it can go into their records. So that is a hurdle that they do not share it with providers, and they try putting up with it themselves.

Another provider explained, this phenomenon on the basis of service member concerns about career advancement, explaining, "If [patients] are on a profile for more than two days, what do they do with the uniform, right? So culturally, that puts us at a disadvantage." Additional providers shared challenges stemming from their perception of patients not being forthcom-ing about how the pain initially started and its full severity.

Relatedly, staff (n = 10; administrators = 2, providers = 8) discussed potential impacts of pain treatment on service members being marked as "not deployable" or losing their military position or special status (e.g., flight status or special operations status). In some cases, pro-viders observed that patient concerns about deployability or losing special status were a bar-rier to them seeking care. For example, one provider stated,

> You see lots of guys who were rangers, ops [operations] in special forces for years, and you never see them until they're 38 or 45 years old and getting ready to retire and have all these pain complaints because they didn't want to be taken out of their career or taken off-duty or become nondeployable.

Providers also remarked that periods of being nondeployable because of taking certain medi-cations were perceived by some patients to harm their chances at career progression in the military. A provider explained, "nobody wants to be grounded. So it's a barrier to [patients] not making an accurate complaint or statement of what's actually going on. Like, they don't want a profile. I think they hold back about [their pain]." Providers also acknowledged that medical evaluation board requirements complicated pain treatment. Said one provider, "Learning the med board [medical evaluation board] stuff, everything that comes along with having an active-duty patient. It can be complicated."

Unavailability of Treatments and Poor Appointment Availability

Some staff ($n = 20$; administrators = 4, providers = 16) also discussed the unavailability of treatments, including pain management and other specialty services. Providers at MTFs with no pain management clinic identified this as an access barrier, and pain management providers pointed to the limited capacity of their clinic as a challenge. In an example of the latter, a pain management provider stated, "So, ten [pain management] providers isn't actually enough for the volume that we have. We're running a very efficient clinic. There also isn't enough capacity in [the MTF metro area] in the community to take care of all of our patients." Other providers who discussed access barriers remarked more generally on "not having the resources" they needed. For example, one provider offered, "Like most places I've been, we have a lot of people who try hard to provide good services, but at some point, you are limited by resources." Staff also discussed barriers stemming from the lack of TRICARE reimbursement for some treatments when provided in community-based settings that might assist with pain care. One administrator and one provider also mentioned geographic distance to health services as a barrier to care for patients.

Staff ($n = 20$; administrators = 4, providers = 16) discussed barriers related to poor appointment availability. Two administrators discussed a lack of appointments, and one raised the long waiting period for pain management clinics. Four providers similarly discussed a lack of appointments; one stated,

> Chronic pain patients require a lot of time and effort for different issues. Usually there is not one issue. It's the pain, the impact, the psychological factors, medication management, and so forth. The only way to take care of them is to see them more frequently. You can tell them to come back. But if there are no appointments, you do the best you can.

Providers also discussed waiting times being too long and, in a couple of cases, causing active-duty patients to seek care off-base.

Challenges with Patient Engagement and Expectations

Some staff ($n = 15$; administrators = 0, providers = 15) discussed issues related to patient preferences and perceptions, including some patients' lack of buy-in to engage in care or accept clinical recommendations. Providers highlighted a lack of patient readiness to engage in pain treatment, low adherence to medications, and noncompliance with treatment plans. Two providers felt that some patients displayed distinct mindsets: one, an attitude of "no pain, no gain," and the other, a desire for treatment convenience. Others discussed unrealistic patient expectations as a challenge.

Provider Challenges Accessing Training

Another common barrier highlighted by staff ($n = 14$; administrators = 5, providers = 9) was difficulty accessing pain care–related training. These staff also described existing trainings as difficult to access and implement. Explained one administrator, "I think what's been more helpful for providers is training opportunities. But for one, those can be very difficult to come by, and two, we have so many other requirements for our active-duty officers, [so] to let them go for training opportunities is sometimes difficult." Another administrator acknowledged that pain champions receive protected training time, but stated, "there's kind of really no other set protected time for any provider [to attend meetings or receive pain care training]." One provider acknowledged barriers to training, stating, "If it's somewhere they have to send you, then you're talking money . . . your schedule having to be covered by somebody else to allow you to get the training, so it becomes a little difficult."

Challenges with Electronic Health Records

Another barrier discussed by staff (n = 14; administrators = 3, providers = 11) was related to the EHR. Some generally spoke of a lack of efficiency of their existing EHR. One provider expanded on their experience of using AHLTA,

> The [EHR] is completely inefficient. It takes me a while to document anything. There are different ways of pain assessment and there are notes that [somebody] just developed and may or may not have an idea of what a pain assessment is, what is DoD-mandated based off of clinical practice guidelines, but it's there. It provides, it gets information, but does not import relevant information. It is not efficient. . . . I'm spending a disproportionate amount of time documenting and trying to figure out what has already been done rather than trying to treat the patient in front of me.

At the time of the interviews, MTFs were in various stages of transition to the adoption of the new EHR platform MHS GENESIS; some MTFs were using GENESIS and others were still utilizing the older system, AHLTA. At least one provider mentioned frequent system outages or failures associated with AHLTA. An administrator and a few providers highlighted challenges stemming from lack of familiarity with navigating GENESIS. One provider mentioned its tendency to "fail" or become unavailable to use.

Other Barriers

Other barriers cited by staff members are described here.[7]

Challenges with Care Coordination and Continuity

Staff (n = 7; administrators = 1, providers = 6) also discussed challenges with care coordination and continuity of care. Providers reported challenges tracking and coordinating care for patients receiving pain care from TRICARE providers in the community. One primary care provider remarked, "Sometimes they do get pushed to the civilian side, which makes it hard to follow the care, just because our EMR [electronic medical record] is not the same." Providers and administrators alike discussed barriers to continuity of care; one provider stated, "I

---

[7] Barriers discussed here were discussed by fewer than 15 percent of staff members and were not thematically related to one of the aforementioned barriers that *were* discussed by at least 15 percent of staff members.

see a lot of [different] patients, unless I say specifically, 'Please come back and see me in one month.' I think pain patients need consistency."

Provider Inexperience with Pain Care

Several staff ($n = 5$; administrators = 1, providers = 4) also raised provider inexperience as a barrier. Notably, the administrator shared that residents and physicians typically do not receive formal education on treating chronic pain. Two providers expressed challenges associated with treating a military population without having personal experience with military service, thereby limiting knowledge of military medicine and terminology. One provider also shared personal challenges with treating chronic pain:

> I think if I'm honest, I don't really love treating pain, so . . . I'm not as adventurous or inquisitive about the newest techniques and actively searching the literature for new ideas to have a certain set of tools that I use. . . . And as much as [I] want to try to figure out and get to the bottom of what is causing someone's pain, sometimes, I just am not that interested.

Unit- or Command-Related Barriers

In addition, some staff ($n = 4$; administrators = 0, providers = 4) also highlighted unit- or command-related barriers, including the consequential impacts of a lack of commander buy-in and of a unit not following clinical guidance, potentially worsening a service member's pain outcome. One staff member commented,

> The commanders not buying into their treatment plan [is a barrier]. The leadership. If I put a patient on a profile, my things are only recommendations . . . and [if] their commander or leadership is like, "No, you're still going to do these things because that is just a recommendation on the profile," the commander can override everything.

Patient Perceptions of Barriers to Care

Patients ($n = 54$) were asked whether anything had gotten in the way of their pain care. Most patients were probed on specific barriers, including finding a provider or where to get care, appointment availability and wait times, getting to appointments (e.g., away from duties and travel time), cost, and stigma.[8] Here, we present the most common barriers to care for patients.

---

[8] Unlike with staff interviews, we asked patients about barriers at only one point in the interview (i.e., we did not ask patients to identify barriers specific to opioid prescribing or NPT). Thus, although we discussed staff barriers in three separate chapters (barriers of appropriate opioid prescribing in Chapter 5, barriers to provider use of NPT in Chapter 6, and overarching barriers to good pain care in Chapter 7), patient barriers are discussed in this chapter only.

Lack of Available Appointments

Over half of patients ($n = 36$) stated that a lack of available appointments was a barrier to their care. Sometimes patients attributed long wait times for specialty appointments to the limited number of providers available. This sentiment was also true for primary care. Patients reported that it felt "impossible to get care" in specific regions because appointments were booked out for "three, four, five months." One patient stated, "The ability to schedule and receive treatment for any particular treatment seems to be an arduous journey. . . . Whether you're trying to use the walk-in hours or you're trying to schedule it through a provider." Patients described their frustration in scheduling two weeks to a few months out, and one stated, "[When] you're living with pain, it's two weeks to a month of misery. So that's a little frustrating." Another explained, "You could legit feel like . . . something is really going on with something in your body, or something just say that's really bothering you, [and] you might not get seen for maybe, you know, a month. Like here, it's up to a month." With regard to specialty care, one patient mentioned that there was only one practicing chiropractor in the local area, which, in turn, made it very difficult to schedule an appointment. He stated,

> I have a friend of mine who also has back problems, and he's navigating his way through the system. I had conversation with him, and told I was going to [a] chiropractor. And he was like, "Man you were really lucky, I heard it was really hard to get in to see them." So, there's just not enough [chiropractors].

In addition to challenges faced in scheduling routine primary care and specialty care for chronic pain, patients described challenges with appointment availability for more-urgent issues, such as episodes of acute pain symptoms. For example, one patient said he was forced to seek treatment for his pain in the emergency room because of barriers to outpatient care:

> It's hard to schedule appointments, especially being able to schedule to see a doctor, you have to schedule three to four days out. And it's like, I don't want to have to go to the ER [emergency room]. It's not a bad thing, but the only thing [ER providers] do is try to stop the overall initial pain, and from there, you need to get scheduled [for continued care]. But sometimes that pain is not manageable for those few days [i.e., the three to four days it takes to schedule], and you have to still go to work. And then when you do come in [for the appointment], it feels like it's very quick, and they just give you what they want to give you. When you do have questions, it's more of a kind of—what's the word—they kind of beat around the bush for it, instead of answering your question initially. Or they'll say they'll get back with you, and they really don't.

Another patient described an instance in which their pain was "so bad I couldn't walk," explaining, "I tried to schedule an appointment, [and] I was told the earliest appointment was a month away. For anything. And [I] was able to get in sooner than that with lots of persistence. But [I] was basically told I could go to the emergency department, or I could wait until they had an appointment."

Speaking to appointment availability more broadly, other patients described scenarios in which it was hard to get ahold of someone on the phone to schedule appointments and having to call back several times. Scheduling appointments was described by one patient as a "nightmare." A patient elaborated on the scheduling difficulties he experienced,

> So, I think that is the biggest issue from the start, the fact that individual shops don't have direct numbers or they don't give it out willy-nilly, so you have to sort of go through a minefield of automated jargon to try and get what you're looking for. And even if you call through that appointment line or whatever, through that automated system, it transfers you over and may actually call a facility, but you don't know what the number is. So, if they don't pick up or if they're at lunch or training day or whatever, you have to navigate that whole process again. Because not every work center allows you to leave phone messages. And I Googled to see what unit codes were what, and I tried to find somebody in that shop through the global, but I feel like I should not have to go out of my way to do that if I am trying to seek medical care.

Stigma

When asked about whether stigma was a barrier that had gotten in the way of receiving pain care, some patients ($n = 18$) indicated that it had. One patient detailed,

> I would throw in the stigma. For example, if you have to leave work, "Why? You left yesterday." And if you can do it all okay in a little bit, you're okay; otherwise, they're like, what's wrong with you? Also in the military, you have to advocate for a waiver in the physical training, and that's its own stigma because a lot of people have knowledge of that. And it's basically a piece of paper saying you can't do something.

Patients also spoke of certain people in their unit who saw physical therapy as a sign of "weakness." One patient recalled being chastised for going to the hospital to go "swimming in the pool" (a part of their physical therapy treatment plan). The patient shared, "So, no [I] don't want to speak about it; people in my unit will see me as weak, and I don't want people to see me like that. I'd rather muscle through and pretend everything's okay. Stigma plays a large part, honestly." Another patient spoke of how seeking treatment for pain was seen as a form of weakness:

> The military is an organization or institution where you cannot demonstrate any type of weakness. But particularly, I will speak for the Army. I don't know about branches, but I suspect that they probably have the same attitude. You cannot demonstrate any type of weakness. And most especially if you are a leader, you definitely cannot demonstrate weakness. Frequent visits to the treatment care facility could be construed as a weakness, and for that reason, there was a lot of time I just stayed away from it. Especially if I had soldiers or people under my charge out there. I don't want to be seen at the treatment facility with soldiers I'm leading because they would probably be like, "Huh, that's my First Sergeant. He's at the hospital too," so there's just a stigma to it. And people deal with whatever

issues that they have, and because they're not getting seen with it or seen for those issues, those issues over time become worse. And by the time they perhaps muster enough courage to seek treatment, the damage may have been done.

One patient remarked, "people look at [people with frequent medical appointments] a little weird sometimes," because "any health condition that gets you away from the job [is stigmatized]." Others cited that unsupportive leadership that perpetuated stigma:

> It's worse for pain. In the past, not in recent years, in the past, I've had issues where you would get cursed out by your leaders because you visited the treatment facility, "What are you looking for over there," you know, those kind of questions, and then they would say, "Get back to work," stuff like that and you just have that mentality, if I'm hurting, if I feel sick, I just have to drag on, I just gotta move on, it'll be fine. And that's just the culture. That is military culture. It could be something wrong with it, but it's just the culture. Because that culture also translates to you being resilient, even in the face of danger when you are dealing with certain types of people in certain types of environment. So, it can work against itself, in a way, [but also], it can help. Because even when you are dealing with pain, you still have the courage, and you still have the resiliency to move on.

Another explained the role of military culture:

> If you end up going to the doctor's, you are considered soft, or something like that sort. That you can't handle it. Even though you have this insurance and a treatment facility here to help you. They make you feel like you shouldn't go, and if you do go, it has to be the worst of the worst before [going]. They make you feel like it has to be a 9 or a 10 before you go, and if it's not, it doesn't really matter. And they'll kind of joke about it. The only thing they won't joke about or stop joking about, is suicide stuff; they will still joke about mental health stuff. It's kind of upsetting.

Patients also spoke of being accused of malingering or "faking their pain" and receiving pushback from providers. One patient shared an anecdote in which a provider took their pain seriously only after seeing the gravity of disease on an MRI.

Those in leadership positions, such as officers, remarked on how their rank was a barrier to care and contributed to stigma. A patient explained, "A lot of the times, being an officer in a hospital or clinic is like wow, they're here, they shouldn't be here, they should be somewhere else. This is for soldiers, but there's like a stigma around officers taking care of themselves." Rank also affected care seeking; the time commitment of pain treatment, such as pain management classes, affected a service member's ability to rise in ranks:

> So if I were to go to that program [in the pain management clinic—the one that requires a lot of time commitment], they would remove me from becoming a platoon leader, which is like the leader in the spot [squad/squadron], in order for me to become a captain. So that's one of the reasons why I wouldn't be able to do that. I have to wait until after pla-

toon leader time, which is about a year, so that's one of the reasons, you know, I guess the stigma in the Army is missing work to go to the health appointments.

Some patients shared how they managed stigma. One patient explained that they were getting over the stigma presented with pain care because, "I get older, I care a little less. I want to get my pain taken care of. I feel like I'm trying to take care of myself a little better." Another stated,

> That [stigma] used to really bother me. But I recently tried to get out and didn't . . . after that and realizing how much me being there did or did not make a difference, at the end of the day, I am very easily replaceable. I kinda decided after I reenlisted after going through all of that that I need to worry about myself too. So it doesn't really bother me anymore because I don't let it. And I try to advocate for my other soldiers that have problems. That you need to take care of yourself.

Difficulty Finding a Provider and Where to Get Care

Patients ($n = 15$) also indicated that they faced barriers to finding a provider or where to get care. The perceived reasons for this were varied and were sometimes not mentioned. However, among those patients who did elaborate, patients discussed high demand and a lack of staff. One patient said, "I feel like they're very undermanned for the amount of [patients] that are coming in and out."

Other patients also mentioned that it was challenging to navigate how to get care. A patient described his experience after a low back injury:

> In September or early October, I kind of stumbled my way around [the MTF], and I was able to talk to the person at the information desk after having tried to call the hotline several times and just getting voice mails. And so I kind of stumbled my way around the [MTF] Clinic for probably two or three hours trying to find the right office for back pain, and then they finally referred me to the [DO]. . . . I wandered around [this MTF] for half a day just trying to find an office that would help me treat back pain.

Another stated, "Trying to reach anyone at the medical facility at [the MTF] is the hardest thing I've tried in my military career."

Additionally, patients also described their lack of a consistent PCM, resulting in greater communication delays and confusion about where to go to receive pain care. One stated,

> I believe it was like last week and a half ago where I said this individual was my PCM, and someone over the phone mentioned they were no longer working there. I'm like, "Oh well, that's good to know." I wish I knew that. It's not like the PCM that was assigned to me, I never met in person, nor have I ever spoken with this PCM. It's always been a different PCM handling my case, which is not a problem because I'm being seen, but it feels like—I mean, everyone should be treated special, but at the same time, it feels like I was being passed around and saying hey, this guy has an issue, PCM we assigned you is not there,

so we'll find another PCM to hear you out. That's pretty much what I've experienced this entire time. I don't know who my PCM is at this point.

Another elaborated by stating, "Yeah, I don't know who my [primary care] provider is. I haven't heard from my provider. I was told I had a total of three to four providers, but I've never seen them. So, it's kind of like, I really—the only care I know to go to is the ER, and that's the best I could do." For patients who did not have a current PCM, it could be challenging to make an appointment to establish care with a new one and even more challenging to get a referral.

Difficulty Getting to Appointments

Some patients ($n = 14$) also described challenges getting away from their military duties or arranging transportation to attend scheduled appointments. Patients mentioned that most appointments were during work hours, requiring them to leave in the middle of a shift: "So you have to come in the middle of your shift, drive a half hour each way, go to the appointment, and 30 minutes to come back. It's not really something that supervisors are into." Intense training regimes imposed even more barriers. As one patient explained,

> A lot of it, for me at least, from stories I've heard, it's really hard to slow down, because my mentality is if I'm slowing down, I'm not fighting, and if I'm not fighting, we're losing. It's a big obstacle, me getting help. If I feel like, oh my back hurts, but they need me on this mission I'm going to just bite the bullet, try to muscle throughout it, but also gets in my way of [the mission].

Commuting time, especially for off-base referrals, was another barrier to treatment. Travel times to get to clinics ranged from an hour to nearly three hours. One patient stated, "I have to write off at least half a day from work to come out here, because hour plus drive there, hour plus appointment, hour plus back, I have to miss at least half a day of work." Another explained, "My care for my back is not on the same base I serve on, so if I've got an appointment for pain management, I have to travel 45 minutes to an hour to get to the pain management clinic, which is very difficult for my schedule."

Other Barriers to Pain Care

This section provides more detail on other barriers discussed by patients.[9]

Technology and System Challenges

Several patients ($n = 4$) cited other barriers to pain care, such as technology and system challenges (e.g., "The provider said all systems were down, so they couldn't order any X-rays; they couldn't order the medicine").

---

[9] Barriers discussed here were cited by fewer than 15 percent of patients and were not thematically related to one of the aforementioned barriers that *were* cited by at least 15 percent of patients.

Cost of Pain Care

Only a few patients ($n = 3$) mentioned that cost was a barrier to their care. Those who did generally discussed difficulties getting access to pain care that was not available at the MTF. For example, patients reported paying out of pocket for massages or chiropractic care because that was sometimes not available on base, or they were referred out to a civilian provider. Another patient remarked on the indirect costs of seeking care in relation to rising gas prices, remarking that "they're not paying me to drive [to appointments]. Gas is five dollars a gallon, and I have to drive a half hour to get gas because there is no gas station on my base."

Lack of Provider Time During Appointments

Additionally, a few patients ($n = 3$) stated that they felt that their providers did not always take the time to listen or did not take their reports of pain seriously (e.g., "Whenever I see a doctor, sometimes they don't want to engage and will be busy").

Barriers Related to the COVID-19 Pandemic

A few patients ($n = 2$) also mentioned the fact that the COVID-19 pandemic changed the dynamic of care and exacerbated existing barriers. For example, a few patients disliked that, as a result of COVID-19, many pain treatments and appointments switched to telehealth. One patient explained that they missed the ability to go in person to physical therapy, remarking that, for the past year, he had "just been given little handouts and bands [for physical therapy]. And they go, 'Okay, go try it at home and good luck, hopefully that works.' Aside from that, it's been [a] very hands off approach for the past year." Also because of COVID-19-related social distancing and limited capacity in clinics, patients said that there were fewer appointments available in a day. A patient summarized, "It's the military; everyone is busy, overworked, and underpaid."

Summary

In this chapter, we described themes from interviews with staff (administrators and providers) and patients with respect to facilitators and strengths as well as barriers to the treatment of service members with chronic pain.

- **Strengths and facilitators of care:** Staff highlighted a myriad of facilitators to providing effective pain treatment. The most commonly cited facilitators were adequate provider training, access to consultation with pain care specialists and other specialty providers, and provider experience. Other facilitators included consultation with pain care champions, consultation with clinical pharmacists, and on-site or nearby access to effective treatments (including pain management clinics and specialty care). Some staff also mentioned the role of nurses or ancillary staff. Relatedly, nearly all patients described one or more strengths or positive aspects of pain care. The most common were having received effective pain treatment and having providers who listened and whose care was patient centered. Some patients reported having good access to treatment options or availability of appointments or having confidence in their providers' ability to accurately diagnose and treat their pain.

- **Barriers to care:** Staff identified multiple barriers to delivering or overseeing pain care; the most common being inadequate appointment length to effectively manage patients with chronic pain, inadequate staffing, military-related issues, and unavailability of some pain treatments and programs. Military-related issues included the stigma often associated with seeking pain care, lack of support for time to engage in treatment, and the fear that receipt of pain care and the related time away from duties may negatively affect a service member's career progression. Similarly, most patients we queried also discussed numerous barriers to receiving pain care. Over half of patients reported long wait times for appointments. Additionally, some patients described other issues, such as stigma associated with seeking pain care, challenges with finding a provider, or difficulty getting to an appointment.

CHAPTER 8

Staff and Patient Recommendations

In this chapter, we summarize recommendations from staff (administrators and providers) and patients on how to improve care for service members with acute and chronic pain. Specifically, we present the recommendations made by staff for overcoming barriers to the delivery of evidence-based care and patient-identified areas of improvement for pain care.

Interviewee Recommendations

We asked staff whether they had recommendations to overcome the barriers they identified as getting in the way of delivering evidence-based pain care. In our conversations with patients, we asked how patients thought pain care could be improved at the MTF. We summarize the responses of both staff and patients. In each category, the results are presented from the most to least endorsed.[1] Figure 8.1 provides an overview of the most common recommendations endorsed by staff and patients.

Staff Recommendations to Overcome Barriers to Delivering Evidence-Based Pain Care

Staff (*n* = 68; administrators = 15, providers = 53) were asked to provide recommendations that they felt might address the barriers to delivering evidence-based pain care. There were no specific follow-up probes. Some shared insights reflect general recommendations made by staff throughout the discussions.

Hire More Staff

Staff provided recommendations to address perceived staffing shortages and challenges with retention (*n* = 34; administrators = 7, providers = 27). They suggested hiring additional providers across a breadth of specialties or offering higher pay to support retention. A provider emphasized the need for more staff, suggesting that the MHS "just hire[s] enough people to do the job. Being able to help [leadership] understand the value of what our team does. We

---

[1] Recommendations that are thematically similar are grouped into one report heading or category. The recommendation in each category that was endorsed by the largest number of respondents is what determines the overall order of that category in the report.

FIGURE 8.1

Recommendations Endorsed by Staff and Patients

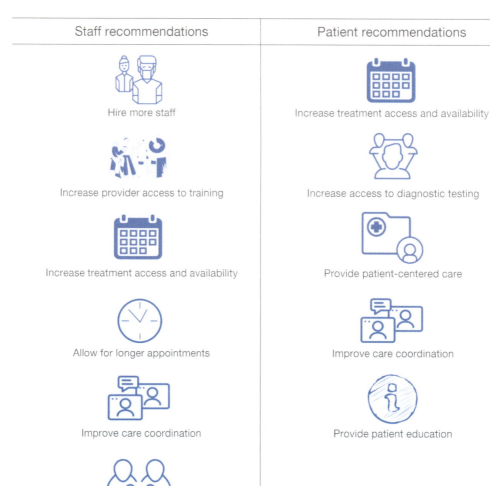

Staff recommendations	Patient recommendations
Hire more staff	Increase treatment access and availability
Increase provider access to training	Increase access to diagnostic testing
Increase treatment access and availability	Provide patient-centered care
Allow for longer appointments	Improve care coordination
Improve care coordination	Provide patient education
Increase patient engagement	

NOTE: The figure includes recommendations endorsed by 15 percent or more staff members (N = 68) and those endorsed by 15 percent or more patients (N = 54).

should not be hampered by not having enough staff." An administrator highlighted the need to provide adequate compensation, stating, "I feel when you have discrepancy from sister services [VA and DoD], we're at a competitive disadvantage to retaining talent. It really needs to be a realistic pay scale; you can't really have an [acupuncturist] be a tech-level GS [General Schedule]-7 or -8 when VA will put them at a [GS]-10 or -11." A couple of providers also recommended that consideration be placed on balancing the appropriate number of patients per staff member. Relatedly, some staff (*n* = 8; administrators = 1, providers = 7) discussed the need for additional nursing and ancillary staff; most providers highlighted a need for a greater number of nurses.

Increase Provider Access to Training

Some staff ($n = 22$; administrators = 5, providers = 17) recommended provider training. Specifically, administrators recommended changes to CME credits and increasing the number and types of CME trainings available. One administrator also recommended rotation of the pain champion presenter at the Project ECHO sessions to encourage specialized skills development among attendees. Relatedly, three providers also spoke of Project ECHO sessions, both encouraging they be better advertised to increase uptake. Other providers recommended the provision of more-general training on specialty services, such NPT as battlefield acupuncture, and pain management. Said one primary care provider,

> As I said, I am lucky to get trained in acupuncture. I don't know how other people get the opportunity. . . . I just feel I have more choices for the patient [since] I learned acupuncture. Now I can have a totally different approach. As opposed to the past, [when] I would them [patients] to pain management and follow whatever [pain management specialists] need me to do. . . . I think we just need a little more training. . . . That would be very helpful. I think that would facilitate more [use of] nonpharmaceutical [treatment], instead of opioids, which is now becoming more and more hard to prescribe without worrying about all the consequences and side effects of it.

Said another primary care provider, "Training would be nice, like we already talked about. I think the off-site [training] would be a good opportunity to get someone from the [nearby MTF] pain clinic down here [to facilitate training]."

A few staff ($n = 3$; administrators = 1, providers = 2) recommended working with health professionals other than doctors—such as physician assistants or nurse practitioners—to help increase provider awareness of available resources for pain care or to share some of the work. One provider recommended the use of visiting pain specialists to help increase connections between different providers in the clinic, whereas the other spoke of increasing provider awareness about new medications for pain care. The latter explained, "We have utilized Marinol [cannabinoid] with game-altering, life-altering success compared to anything else I've ever prescribed [for pain]. So, getting more knowledge out there, getting more of the medical community aware."

Increase Treatment Access and Availability

Increasing access to and availability of treatments was discussed by over one-third of staff ($n = 25$; administrators = 4, providers = 21); one provider stated, "Well, I mean, the main thing is to improve or increase the possibility to offer more [treatment] choices to the patient." Administrators discussed increasing the number of specialty services offered, including physical medicine and rehabilitation, acupuncture, chiropractic manipulation, and medical massage, and having clinics available that are solely dedicated to treating musculoskeletal concerns among active-duty patients. Relatedly, providers suggested increasing access to specialty services including acupuncture, chiropractic care, and physical therapy. One provider encouraged a focus on preventive services that might mitigate pain severity.

Some staff ($n = 7$; administrators = 2, providers = 5) offered recommendations regarding appointment scheduling and strategies for addressing limited appointment availability. As a stopgap measure for dealing with appointment delays, the administrator suggested communicating pain self-management strategies that the patient might utilize in the interim while waiting for their referral appointment to occur. The providers recommended extending office hours beyond the business day or allowing flexibility in scheduling multiple follow-up and referral appointments at once. One provider suggested offering NPT, such as BH interventions, in group rather than individual sessions to increase appointment availability. Another provider recommended bringing certain specialty services into clinics to reduce wait times associated with referrals.

Allow for Longer Appointments

Staff ($n = 14$; administrators = 3, providers = 11) recommended that appointments for chronic pain patients be longer, citing the need for adequate time to explain or administer treatments and manage more-complex patient cases. An administrator offered two suggestions to implement such a recommendation: "have the flexibility to make those [primary care visits] longer visits or double book, back-to-back, so that you can really give those [complex] patients the depth of care that they require." A primary care provider explained, "I would say [having] 30 minutes [for appointments] as opposed to 20 minutes would be huge in primary care. Our subspecialists get 30- to 60-minute appointments to deal with one issue, and we have to deal with a dozen in one 20-minute visit."

Improve Care Coordination

Furthermore, staff ($n = 11$; administrators = 2, providers = 9) recommended improvements to care coordination, communication between providers, and care continuity. An administrator cited as an example the new Air Force initiative for PCMs that dedicates protected time toward review of patient profiles and histories. Providers suggested ideas that, in some cases, overlapped with other recommendations pertaining to staffing or provider awareness. For example, they suggested preventing lapses in care broadly through the hiring of nursing and ancillary staff, such as nurse case managers; making it easier for providers to learn about available treatments; and empowering PCMs to engage in "specialty coordination" of pain care patients. One provider explained, "If DHA is looking at how could we improve monitoring and communication and tracking, if you had a nurse case manager or an RN [registered nurse] or a designated person for each team . . . then things wouldn't get missed."

Increase Patient Engagement

Staff ($n = 11$; administrators = 3, providers = 8) suggested strategies for increasing patient engagement, such as through outreach to service members to encourage them to seek care and patient education on what chronic pain is and which treatment modalities are appropriate. For example, one provider recommended, "Patient education, number one. In order to have better patient education and get patient buy-in, we need longer appointment times . . . to set realistic expectations for pain and get patient buy-in." In describing their suggestions for outreach to service members, one provider recommended, "taking . . . preventative strategies out to the squadron to kind of educate them before a chronic pain situation develops." Another provider suggested, "More education to the service members in general about seeking care. [Seeking pain care] doesn't make them weaker; it makes them smarter."

Other Recommendations

The following additional recommendations were endorsed by MTF staff.[2]

Support Specialty Pain Clinics

Some staff (n = 9; administrators = 5, providers = 4) made recommendations regarding specialty pain clinics or programs, with all discussing the IPMCs and some suggesting that their funding be better protected by DoD. An administrator emphasized, "I would implore Congress, the Pentagon, [and] DoD: Please restore allocated funds for IPMCs and prevent them from being utilized by commands for other purposes other than staffing the IPMCs directly." One primary care provider suggested allocating resources for pain management clinics proportional to the number of service members with chronic pain at an MTF rather than the overall size of the MTF.

Improve Decision Support

Staff (n = 6; administrators = 3, providers = 3) recommended improved EHR or decision support. Staff at MTFs still using AHLTA suggested improving the reliability of the EHR and the quality of available decision support tools.[3] One provider stated, "It sounds like they're giving us GENESIS. I don't know if it'll make it better or worse; we'll see." Another explained:

> If I see a patient and AHLTA is down, and if I have a chronic pain patient who I've never seen [before], you cannot rely on a patient to be an awesome historian of what they've received and what they've done. That never happens. Having reliable systems that work 100 percent of the time [is necessary]. I understand 100 percent is not feasible, but at least better systems that help us as providers to utilize our plan of care.

Staff at MTFs using GENESIS suggested improving alerts and allowing for "agility in our templating" to support scheduling longer visits. An administrator recommended that the alert to consider prescribing naloxone for at-risk patients should have a "one-click button to

---

[2] Recommendations discussed here were endorsed by fewer than 15 percent of staff members and were not thematically related to one of the aforementioned recommendations that *were* endorsed by at least 15 percent of staff members.

[3] At the time of our interviews, MTFs were at different stages in the transition from AHLTA to the new EHR system, MHS GENESIS.

prescribe the Narcan right there on that warning page" rather than requiring that providers close the alert and navigate multiple additional screens.

Modify DHA Policy or Operations

Staff ($n = 6$; administrators = 2, providers = 4) also made recommendations for changing DHA policy or operations more broadly. For example, an administrator suggested that DHA take a more "hands-off" approach and allow MTFs to guide decisionmaking and practice with respect to pain care at the local level: "I think leadership should put out general guidance. Don't flood MTFs with a thousand taskings, and trust us to do our jobs. And when you do that, I think you generally get a good result." Providers advocated for increased DHA leadership support for pain management. One provider recommended changes to improve care delivery, suggesting funding a revision of the Joint Pain Education Program to ensure that it is up to date. Notably, one provider reinforced their other recommendation of using "DoD health care dollars" to increase access to NPT provided off-base, remarking, "Our [existing] system—we don't necessarily incentivize getting better. We incentivize getting worse and getting out, so changing some of those policies would probably help too."

Revise Referral Requirements

In addition, several staff ($n = 4$; administrators = 1, providers = 3) highlighted referral practice–related recommendations. The administrator suggested that patients be referred to pain care earlier in the course of their care to allow adequate time to receive a course of NPT before a deployment or permanent change of station. Two providers recommended increasing access to physical therapy, although one suggested doing so by removing the referral requirement from primary care (i.e., allowing for self-referral), whereas the other suggested referring earlier and more often to physical therapy and sports medicine. Another provider, who perceived that DHA recommended that "anyone that has pain need to see a psychologist," also recommended that the DHA revisit this referral guidance given perceived barriers in access to BH care for patients experiencing BH conditions.

Other Treatment-Related Recommendations

Several staff ($n = 4$; administrators = 1, providers = 3) offered treatment-related recommendations. One provider recommended moving away from narcotic medications in treating chronic pain given their lack of effectiveness and advocated for use of NPT and exercise, whereas another provider encouraged the infusion of traditional medicine (e.g., Mediterranean diet) into Western practices.

Unit- or Command-Related Recommendations

Finally, a few staff ($n = 3$; administrators = 0, providers = 3) discussed unit- or command-related recommendations. Two providers from separate MTFs suggested embedding a medic in each unit, though for different reasons. One provider suggested that embedded medics could take proactive steps to "try to correct ergonomic issues so that they don't become chronic pain," and another suggested that medics should facilitate communication about pain care between the medical team and command. A third provider suggested providing

PCMs with "administrative time" for communicating with the unit commander about duty restrictions or other aspects of pain care.

Other Organizational Recommendations

A few staff ($n = 2$; administrators = 2, providers = 0) offered other organizational or structural recommendations that DHA might be best positioned to address. An administrator recommended that TRICARE coverage be expanded to cover more off-base NPT, such as chiropractic care or acupuncture, and another recommended that the government ensure supply-chain issues do not result from federal budget discussion standstills.

Patient Recommendations for Pain Care Improvement

We asked all patients ($n = 54$) about their perceptions on how pain care could be improved at their MTF. There were no specific follow-up probes. Most patients ($n = 47$) had specific recommendations for pain care improvement, such as increasing treatment access or appointment availability; increasing access to diagnostic testing; providing patient-centered care; improving the referral process and strengthening care coordination and continuity of care; and providing patient education for the prevention of chronic pain. Other suggestions included changing military culture to reduce stigma and improving systems to communicate with a clinic to schedule or follow up on appointments. Other patients ($n = 7$) offered no recommendations.

Increase Treatment Access and Availability

The most common recommendation made by patients for improving pain care was to increase treatment access or expand availability of appointments. A little over half of patients ($n = 29$) recommended increasing access to treatments that were not available at some MTFs, such as chiropractic care or specialty pain care. As one put it, "Get a chiropractor back. That would help a lot." Another patient stated,

> I think they should give more money to [pain care], because a lot of guys walk around with like jacked-up backs. Like, there's a lot of wear and tear. So investing more money in these [treatments]. . . . Just increase access . . . there are a lot of people out there that don't know [what's out there]. I lived with this [pain] for a while, thinking it was a pain in the butt, either (1) because I was ignorant that there was something that could help it, or (2) I know there would be something to help, but it was going to be so difficult to get help for it.

Patients also commented that expanding TRICARE reimbursement for services received from community providers and referring patients off-post could help increase access to specialty services. One patient stated, "They should be doing referrals, book your soldiers to go off-post and see a civilian doctor." Another mentioned that they wished TRICARE would increase "accessibility to network or outside network providers," particularly in cases where they faced delays seeking care at the MTF. One patient remarked that there should be fewer limits on how often a patient could go to the chiropractor (e.g., one patient said he used up all 12 chiropractic visits at his previous MTF). Another mentioned that more providers and appointments would allow patients to be seen more frequently—and, for patients that travel for work, afford them greater flexibility and appointment access. A patient stated: "If this amount of care [referring to services provided through a pain clinic] would be accessible to everyone, [that] would be great. It just kind of sucks, the amount of hoops I had to jump through to get to this level." Other patients suggested hiring more primary care providers, pain management specialists, or chiropractors. As one patient stated, "Perhaps there's too much administration and not enough providers."

Relatedly, some patients ($n = 22$) emphasized the importance of reducing long wait times for appointments for both primary care and referrals for other treatments. If PCMs are back-logged with appointments, they said, it would take longer to get to the specialty referral to continue their treatment. As one patient explained,

> For a patient to wait three months to get an appointment, to me, that's ridiculous. . . . Because there's a lot of things that hinge on being able to go to an appointment. . . . In the meantime, during these three months, the soldier has to participate in a number of exercises and a number of trainings. And the soldier is probably not going to be able to complete those trainings to the best of their ability because of whatever [pain] conditions that they have. . . . And then, in the process, the soldier probably gets into trouble because the soldier did not give 100 percent [during training exercises]. And it goes downhill from there. . . . Is there an opportunity, which I think there is, [to shorten that waiting period by referring soldiers to network providers]? After all, soldiers are being referred to specialty clinics to see civilian providers. They can do the same thing [for primary care]; either is a long wait time.

Others mentioned that despite being on time for appointments, long waits in crowded wait-ing rooms and backlogged providers affected their ability to be seen in a timely manner.

Additionally, several patients ($n = 5$) described how building time into military training schedules for physical therapy or other pain treatment would be beneficial for increasing access, especially for those with hectic schedules. Certain patients we spoke to had physical therapy embedded in each of their units, which made it more accessible—however, they were still sent home to do their stretches. A patient reported, "I have a problem of actually finding time to do my stretches. Yeah, so if I had like a standing appointment each week or something to do stretches each week, yeah it would remind me better. Because I just forget. I go home and don't do them."

Finally, one patient highlighted the need for strategies to accommodate people traveling to appointments at MTFs far away, such as allowing for some of the previsit work to be done remotely: "I feel like a lot of times they don't take into consideration the fact that we have to travel to come out here, and a lot of time they're not even aware [where] we're coming from. . . . They don't make an effort to allow us to do the paperwork virtually, to let us send it in, stuff like that."

Increase Access to Diagnostic Testing

About one-quarter of patients (n = 13) believed that increased access to diagnostic testing—particularly imaging—would lead to improved pain care. For example, certain patients felt that diagnostic tools, such as MRIs, should be utilized earlier and more often to diagnose the cause of pain. Explained one patient, "Providers are very hesitant to do imaging, so . . . the typical thing is, you do six months of physical therapy before they'll even consider an MRI for something." Another suggested, "Maybe do X-rays and MRIs first, before physical therapy, because you can actually do physical therapy and hurt the issue more without those images telling [the provider] what's actually wrong." One patient further explained, "I've had . . . the same ankle injury on both my ankles where I had torn ligaments. And because I could still walk, they would make me do six months of physical therapy before an MRI. And then they noticed that the ligaments were torn."

Other patients suggested that it should not take weeks, months, or years to receive an MRI or diagnostic imaging if it is requested by the patient early on in treatment. One patient explained the potential implications of *not* adopting improved processes for diagnosis and evaluation, describing a delay that they experienced and how it affected their pain, "It was two months before I got an MRI and they were like, 'Your bulge is ultra-severe and completely smashing your sciatic nerve.'" As another patient with a recent spine injection put it, "[I] went to schedule an MRI so they can get more imaging and tailor my treatment better. . . . I couldn't get an MRI. . . . That's frustrating. That is six, seven weeks I am waiting, living with pain."

However, these patient recommendations may be contrary to CPGs and evidence-based medicine. In many cases, imaging is not recommended or appropriate as part of an initial work-up for pain and may result in worse outcomes and increased cost (Jacobs et al., 2020). Advanced imaging, such as MRIs and CT [computerized tomography] scans, in particular, are recommended only after other treatment failures (e.g., lack of clinical improvement with NSAIDs or physical therapy), with concerning exam findings (e.g., neurologic deficits), in the setting of trauma, or in patients with a history of cancer (Chou et al., 2009; Jacobs et al., 2020; U.S. Department of Veterans Affairs and U.S. Department of Defense, 2022a). The VA/DoD CPG for low back pain advises against routine imaging but makes it clear that imaging is appropriate when progressive or serious neurologic deficits or other red flags are present (U.S. Department of Veterans Affairs and U.S. Department of Defense, 2022a). Therefore, some of these patient recommendations may reflect a deficit in knowledge because of a communication breakdown between patients and providers as to the appropriate use and timing of advanced imaging. They also reflect patient frustration with long appointment wait times associated with these tests when ordered.

Provide Patient-Centered Care

Another common theme was the importance of providers' sharing different treatment options, listening to patients, customizing treatment to a patient's specific needs, and spending more time with the patient.

Some patients (*n* = 11) mentioned that they felt their provider could have done a better job explaining the different options before deciding on a treatment plan with the patient. As one patient commented, "I would definitely say for people with chronic [pain of any kind], instead of trying to overly medicate people, try to figure out what specialty they need, and go to that." Another patient felt like "the doctor goes from patient to patient really fast, and they don't spend quality time that a civilian doctor necessarily would, saying these are your options, versus straight military get it done, get it done." Other patients recommended that providers emphasize "active" treatment options, such as physical therapy, rather than treatments like medications. A patient explained the benefit of stretching techniques and how physical therapy and chiropractic care "have actually worked for me in my life. And just telling me to have ibuprofen and telling my job I won't be at work for a few days hasn't helped. Versus seeing that the stretching and physical therapy was helpful to the body directly. Instead of just masking pain."

Some patients (*n* = 10) recommended that providers listen to and "believe" their patients when they described their condition and pain care needs. They indicated this would be a more deliberate approach to treating their pain rather than what they perceived in some cases as a dismissive or rote response of providers suggesting they take the "physical therapy and take more ibuprofen [NSAID]" route. As one patient put it, "With regard to PCMs, specifically here but I've had others, it tends to be very much a check the box thing. Like okay, okay, go." Others mentioned decreasing the use of telehealth and increasing in-person visits for patients with pain, suggesting they were not feeling heard during telehealth visits. Patients also reported not being taken seriously for their pain when seen in person or having to come in multiple times before they felt their provider listened or recognized their pain. One described,

> The biggest upset was the beginning, coming in and not [being] taken seriously. I had to come back again to be taken seriously. If [there was someone who] wasn't as persistent as me, they might give up, or feel helpless or hopeless. And start spiraling. And if their unit leadership is not supportive, on top of facing the same barriers I faced to accessing pain care, it could be even more challenging. I've been in the military for so long, I know how to navigate through it. But if there's a new Joe off the street, he might not be familiar with it, or the communication.

Additionally, some patients (*n* = 9) suggested that pain care could be improved if providers would customize treatment to the individual patient. In some cases, this recommendation seemed to stem from a feeling that providers did not always take the time to consider the patient's specific situation before advising on treatment. A patient explained, "Try not give people meds, meds, meds [without customizing treatment to individual preferences] . . . meds just mask the situation without actually helping. It's just like a Band-Aid. [I prefer] long-term resolutions . . . for the pain to go away." Another patient stated, "[Providers should provide] specialized [treatment], in terms of really getting to understand what the issue is with a particular patient and scale the level of care to that particular patient. Instead of, in my view, a general approach to providing care." One patient asserted, "if someone keeps coming back with the same problem, I feel like . . . looking deeper into it, would be smart. Being better at identifying chronic issues [is important], and there's some really bad attitudes in the health area of this base."

Lastly, some patients ($n = 7$) discussed the need for longer appointments to allow time to adequately address patient concerns and develop a treatment plan. A patient advised that providers "get more personal interaction [with patients] versus, 'get them in, get them out' as fast as possible. That's the biggest one. . . . It would just be taking more time to actually get to know patients." Relatedly, a patient commented on the importance of providers taking the time during the appointment to better understand the patient and their medical history, remarking:

> I think if there was a true fundamental understanding of the patient, [that would be beneficial]. And I know everyone's busy, and I can't tell them how to do their job . . . but it could be helpful for them to maybe get into the patient's chart and kind of understand, what have they been through, what has been tried on them? . . . Even as we go through the survey [these questions], even right now, as I'm speaking with you, I'm recalling things that, oh gosh, I forgot to tell you that. Now, imagine 15 minutes with provider, I'm not going to remember all things [to tell them]. It's incumbent on them to look through [the patients'] charts to see what's been done and [ensure adequate] marketing and communicating additional resources to everyone. . . . I don't know how many times I've been [at clinic MTF], but every single time I leave I go, I don't think they've seen my file. That's what I would say that could be improved.

Improve Care Coordination

Patients also underscored the need for better patient follow-up and referral coordination, care continuity, and communication between providers. The most common recommendation was to improve management of referrals and establish processes for following up with patients ($n = 11$). This suggestion included improving staff follow-up between appointments, ensuring patients followed the treatment plan, or allowing for earlier appointments because of cancellations. As one explained, "We have status updates of dang near everything in the military; we could probably have someone sit with you and say, 'Hey we did a new MRI, and this is what the radiologist thinks. This what we're looking at, this is your goal for April, May."

Several patients ($n = 4$) discussed the need to reduce rates of attrition among providers or improve continuity of care for patients whose military duties interrupted their treatment. Oftentimes, patients would have to relocate because of a permanent change of station, necessitating changing providers. This was a hindrance to their pain care and treatment and its continuity. One patient described the constant change of providers as "difficult." When starting fresh, patients also had to repeat their medical history, which they indicated as tedious and burdensome. A patient explained the benefits of keeping the same provider:

From my own perspective, from somebody that unfortunately has to go in and see a PCM potentially like every 90 days, it would be nicer to be able to see [the] same face and then that same face be able to see my face and understand each time, like OK. I remember this patient. And these are the reasons why we did what we did or this is what's happening with their care now and this is the reason why they're asking for certain treatment kind of thing rather than reintroducing myself in attempting to articulate just what's going on with my body each and every single time all over again.

Relatedly, a few patients ($n = 3$) discussed the need for improved communication between providers. They recommended that providers read their electronic medical records to review their treatment history. One stated, "[It's important for providers to] review records. Because then I get all confused every time, I just repeat myself . . . because I got a lot of things going on . . . and then all the different locations they sent me, and who said what." Others went further, wanting their providers to directly discuss their case with other providers. One patient explained that although he doesn't think his pain care is bad, he wishes his providers were talking to one another more often. After having an experience with civilian providers, he could tell the civilian providers had better communication with each other and the "level of visibility and the level of care, and the control, is greater." Another patient described poor communication between his PCM and mental health provider, which resulted in confusion for him around a medication he was taking. A patient explained the benefits of increased provider-to-provider communication:

I think the moment you get that second modality, there should be some sort of fail-safe, so that the moment that happens, you know, there's forced conversation between the professionals. So, to talk about cases, I'm not sure if that would be prohibitive in some cases, but if you have multiple modality care in one facility, I mean, it's in the same building; they should be able to sit down and talk about it. It seems like they're having that conversation only in pain management [at a nearby MTF] . . . and it seems like they should be having the conversation [here at this MTF, also]."

Lastly, a few patients ($n = 2$) pointed to the need to "improve systems" to ensure that they are able to reach someone at the clinic to schedule appointments or inquire about the status of a referral or diagnostic test.

Provide Patient Education

Patients also mentioned the importance of patient education and outreach to facilitate awareness of resources for prevention and treatment for service members. Some patients ($n = 8$) had recommendations for ways to reengineer certain aspects of pain care to increase awareness of treatment options. For example, one patient stated,

It would be nice to see some changes or some improvements in marketing, advertising, and helping service members with pain management. I could send you guys, 20 to 30 [service members I know] who are trying to deal with pain management for years and are still trying to figure it out. The military has to get better resources to help figure this out [for them]. We need better awareness of options for pain and medical or wellness.

Patients recounted various educational programs at MTFs on topics ranging from weight loss to health and wellness. The same patient further stated,

> I'm thinking, "What else do I not know?" There is probably a pain clinic I'm not aware of. I can't tell you how many emails I get of something being broadcast, and there is hardly anything in regard to medical, pain, or wellness that's out there . . . but what else am I missing?

One patient stated, "With some of these services, I almost wish [there were] recruiting briefs and stuff like that. I almost wish they could do like a recruitment fair, to . . . get their names out there more." He later stated he had some "really phenomenal doctor experiences" and would have never known about it if he wasn't in SOCOM or referred from the main compound.

Patients also spoke highly of and recommended the creation of additional support groups, acknowledging the benefits of such groups for increasing awareness of treatment options and sharing strategies for managing chronic pain. One stated, "There are people who are dedicated to helping me manage this pain, just being told that and seeing that . . . I am supported by people who can relate and people who can help instead of thinking that this is just a me thing." A patient who recommended implementing support groups explained the rationale,

> Having that support group and learning about what's working for different people with chronic pain, whether or not it's helpful, that would be helpful. Or like a knowledge of it: What is pain management? So, we talk about like . . . if a doctor says we do dry needling here, not everyone knows that. So, we don't even know what is available to us unless someone tells us. Because some doctors think you should just take drugs and go to the gym [to treat your pain].

Additionally, other patients ($n = 4$) underscored the importance of teaching service members pain and injury prevention and prehabilitation and rehabilitation exercises for better mobility. A patient elaborated, "Recovery is part of physical training. . . . It would cost the government a lot less money just to keep people healthy while they're in [the military] and not to pay people compensation for their VA [benefits] when they get out." Another service member described the importance of education on fitness and chronic pain management "for life":

> I think maybe education [is a recommendation]. . . . In the Marine Corps, they have Fit for Life. You know, it's like, you want to eat well, exercise, and maybe [they should consider] adding a component of education. Just making sure that there are resources there, and hopefully more resources come, but [emphasizing] the importance of just flexibility and stuff. Cause I hit a period—I was always good with my fitness, but just towards the end of my career, I had some personal stuff going on, and just because I wasn't paying attention

to it, I feel like my physical ailments caught up with me. Because I wasn't doing the things that I normally do.

Patients also recommended approaches focused on ergonomics or other interventions to prevent the root cause of chronic pain. For example, one suggested that providers "look and see what the person is doing in their workspace to figure out why they feel the pain . . . if they have back pain, do they get back pain because they move equipment? Is there any way to get equipment to help them with lifting?" Others emphasized the need to take a longer-term view of service members' health and well-being for pain care. A patient stated,

Over time, if you wear combat gear and you go to combat, it has an extended effect over your [physical] frame. And I've spent a few years over there [in combat], and it just sort of weighs on you. And I've heard that in the [Navy] Seal community, I've heard they were doing this, like some of the other SOF [special operations forces] communities—they would take a long-term view of individuals' care. And I think that would be great, if they could think about that, too. Because our backs are usually like one of the first things to go.

Other Recommendations

One other recommendation endorsed by patients is described here.[4]

Reduce Stigma

Additionally, other patients (n = 4) spoke of the importance of reducing stigma around pain care and helping their unit leadership better understand more about pain. A patient remarked, "You can't be a good supervisor unless you know what a pain journey is." Another stated the importance of encouraging service members to get treated for their pain and letting them know that it is okay to get help, because sometimes they might not have the confidence, knowledge, or resources to take care of themselves.

Summary

In this chapter, we described themes from interviews with staff (administrators and providers) and patients with respect to participant recommendations or areas of improvement for the treatment of service members with acute or chronic pain. Recommendations included the following:

- **Increase treatment access and appointment availability:** The most common staff recommendation emphasized a need for hiring more providers. Better access to treatments

---

[4] Recommendations discussed here were endorsed by fewer than 15 percent of patients and were not thematically related to one of the aforementioned recommendations that *were* endorsed by at least 15 percent of patients.

was the second most cited recommendation among staff. Similarly, over half of patients mentioned needed improvements around increasing access to treatments; some suggested that wait times should be reduced for increased availability of appointments.

- **Allow for longer appointments:** Staff also called for allowing for longer appointments, especially for adequate time to manage more-complex patient cases. Relatedly, some patients discussed the need for longer appointments to allow adequate time for developing a treatment plan and addressing patient questions and concerns.

- **Increase provider access to training:** The third most cited recommendation among staff members was increased access to provider training.

- **Increase patient engagement and provide patient-centered care:** Some staff recommended strategies to increase patient engagement in treatment, such as through patient education about what chronic pain is and which treatments might be appropriate. Perhaps in some circumstances and running counter to CPGs for pain, some patients believed that they should have had earlier access to diagnostic testing, particularly imaging. Patients also mentioned the need for increased patient education and improvements around shifting military culture to diminish the stigma associated with seeking pain care. Some patients also endorsed recommendations for providers related to patient-centered care, such as providers' offering counseling about treatment choices, taking the time to listen to patient concerns, and customizing treatment to the individual patient.

- **Improve care coordination:** Staff also felt that care coordination and continuity were central to the delivery of effective pain care. Staff highlighted a need for more nurse care managers and other support staff to facilitate better care coordination and patient follow-up. Similarly, patients also mentioned the need for improved referral management and follow-up.

CHAPTER 9

Findings and Recommendations

In this report, we presented findings from qualitative interviews with 68 staff who oversee or deliver pain care for service members, along with 54 service member patients with chronic pain, recruited from across seven MTFs. These MTFs were selected to maximize variability in quality of pain care and other characteristics (i.e., presence of a pain clinic and service branch, size, and location). Guided by comprehensive interview guides, our interviews captured perspectives on approaches to care, integration of medication and NPT, and respondent recommendations to improve pain care. In this chapter, we describe the strengths and limitations in our analyses, highlight key findings, and offer recommendations on how outpatient pain care delivered by the MHS could be improved.

Strengths and Limitations

The analyses presented in this report have several strengths. The qualitative interviews covered a wide variety of topics related to chronic pain care, including assessment and treatment, use of medications and NPT, facilitators and barriers to pain care, and recommendations for improved care. We conducted the interviews with various respondents, including administrators who oversee pain care, providers of pain care, and service members who received care for chronic pain in the past six months. Therefore, the interviews provided data from multiple perspectives of experience with pain care from several MTFs and across service branches. These qualitative data provided details of care, such as respondent perceptions about shared decisionmaking, coordination of care across multiple providers, and equity of care, that are not captured in administrative data. We used comprehensive coding of the data, which facilitated detailed qualitative data analyses.

Our analyses also had some limitations. Our interviews were limited to staff and patients at MTFs and, therefore, do not reflect staff or patient input from private-sector care. Similarly, our review of MHS efforts to facilitate the implementation of the stepped-care model (beyond monitoring of opioid prescribing, which includes direct and private-sector prescribers) is limited to direct care. We also did not inquire about referral practices or the transition of care from primary to specialty care settings. We selected several MTFs to recruit staff and patients to maximize variation regarding size, service branch, pain care services, and overall quality of care. However, our respondents were not a representative sample of MTF staff and patients. Instead, our qualitative approach aimed to elucidate variability in experiences and perspectives of our respondents. Points of contact at the selected MTFs identified staff for interviews based on criteria that we provided. We did not analyze data for thematic variation by service branch, staff respondent or provider type, or setting. The majority of staff respondents were located in primary care settings, and we did not attempt to analyze data to identify differences between primary care and other treatment settings. Additionally, we aimed to interview at least one BH provider at each MTF, but IBHCs are typically contractors in the Air Force and Navy, so the only BH providers we interviewed were from Army MTFs.

Furthermore, patients were recruited from waiting areas, often from pain clinics. This recruiting approach likely increased the likelihood of including patients who were engaged in ongoing pain care and experiencing more-severe pain symptoms. Interviewers used structured prompts tailored to each respondent type, but the use of probes (i.e., follow-up questions) could vary across interviews, which could have affected the proportion of respondents mentioning particular topics.

Finally, during our data collection, MTFs were using different EHR systems, and some were actively making the switch from AHLTA to GENESIS at the time of our visit. This could have influenced comments that we received about the EHR (particularly mentions of the EHR as a barrier or facilitator of pain care).

Key Findings

Our interviews with staff and service member patients yielded several findings. In this section, we provide an overview of key findings presented in this report.

Nearly All Providers Agreed That Pain Assessment Was Important to Treatment, Yet Only Half Reported Using a Structured Method

The most common consideration in treatment adjustment mentioned by nearly all providers was the severity of pain symptoms or impact of the pain condition on patient functioning. Although nearly all providers reported using some method for this purpose, only approximately half of providers reported that they used a structured method for assessing impact on functioning, such as the DVPRS or PASTOR. Structured assessment is consistent with the stepped-care model, which aims to return a patient's functioning by adjusting care to the patient's needs over time. Nearly all patients reported that their treatment had been adjusted in the previous six months, and most reported that one or more providers assessed the impact of their pain on their daily activities in some way (i.e., through unstructured or structured means) to make this adjustment. In addition, most patients reported that these assessments were administered at every visit and by all or most of their pain care providers. Although these findings support the implementation of stepped care with regular assessment of patient response and functioning as a basis for treatment adjustment, this is best accomplished using the same structured measure for comparison over time (e.g., DVPRS or PASTOR) rather than unstructured means.

Patients Reported Positive Experiences with Shared Decisionmaking, Care Coordination, and Equitable Care, but There Are Opportunities to Improve Patient Experiences

Nearly all providers endorsed using shared decisionmaking with patients when determining a treatment plan for pain and noted the importance of gaining patient buy-in, providing patients with treatment options, and accounting for patients' interests or goals regarding treatment. Consistent with provider perspectives, most patients cited positive experiences with shared decisionmaking. Specifically, most patients said that they were offered a choice of treatment options, felt that their providers explained the benefits and risks of treatments, and believed that their providers listened to their preferences for treatment. Patients reported less favorable perceptions on coordination of care between their providers. Less than half of patients who had more than one provider for their pain care reported that communication between their providers was adequate. Examples of inadequate communication cited by patients were receipt of conflicting treatment recommendations and lack of test result followup. Although most patients felt that they had been treated equitably, nearly one-quarter of patients felt they had been treated differently because of some aspect of their background. The most common reasons patients believed that they were treated differently related to age and rank.

Most Prescribers Expressed Trepidation About Prescribing Opioids

In keeping with the stepped-care model, most prescribers expressed a reluctance to treat chronic pain with opioids and preferred nonopioid medication or NPT as initial treatment. Oral NSAIDs, anticonvulsants, and antidepressants were among the nonopioid medications that prescribers reported using the most to treat chronic pain. Nearly all prescribers across all MTFs expressed trepidation about opioid prescribing; most cited concerns about the safety or addiction potential of opioid medications. Their levels of confidence in prescribing opioids or managing patients who were already taking opioids varied. Most of these individuals indicated that they were currently providing opioid medication to service members with chronic pain, but most told us that they rarely or never initiated opioids, and others said that they did so only as a last resort. Some said that they were comfortable prescribing opioids only to service members with chronic pain as a bridge or if the prescription was initiated by another provider, and some said they would taper inherited LOT patients off opioids. Prescribers expressed concern about the impact of opioids on service member duties or military career. Others stated that they felt opioids were not an effective treatment for chronic pain. However, inheriting service member patients with chronic pain who were prescribed opioids by another provider was described by some as a challenge, and others stated that they were uncertain about how to appropriately prescribe opioids for chronic pain. Nearly all administrators across all MTFs discussed the availability of training to support providers in appropriate opioid prescribing, most mentioned that providers at their clinic or MTF could consult with a pain care specialist or pain champion about opioid prescribing, and half mentioned the availability of consultation with a clinical pharmacist.

Providers Reported Limited Access as the Biggest Barrier to Increased Use of Nonpharmacologic Treatment

More than half of all patients said that they preferred NPT over medication. However, over three-quarters of staff reported barriers in access to NPT, most describing it as the *biggest* barrier to integrating NPT into chronic pain care. Approximately half of all staff cited inadequate staffing, and nearly half mentioned long appointment wait times as a barrier to NPT services. Relatedly, over half of staff commented how limited staffing contributed to decreased access and increased wait times. Despite these barriers, most providers and administrators reported universal use of NPT with all chronic pain patients. Although access to NPT was among the most common factors considered by providers when integrating NPT, providers also considered patients' preferences, willingness to engage in treatment, and clinical presentation (i.e., the type of pain condition, severity, duration, or impact of pain on functioning). Consistent with analyses of administrative treatment data (Hepner et al., 2022), physical therapy was by far the most reported NPT used for the treatment of chronic pain; nearly all providers endorsed it as an NPT that they used the most often, and most patients reported that they had received physical therapy in the past six months. Some providers emphasized the ease of access to physical therapy compared with other NPT. Furthermore, some providers endorsed frequent use of BH care, chronic pain self-management, chiropractic care, acupuncture, and ice or cold therapy. However, with the exception of chiropractic care, these interventions were less commonly reported by patients.

Staff Reported Training and Treatment Access as the Most Important Facilitators of High-Quality Pain Care, Whereas Patients Found Effective Treatment and Patient-Centered Care Most Important

When asked about facilitators to delivering evidence-based pain care, staff most often cited provider training, provider access to consultation with pain care specialists and other specialty providers, and provider experience. Some staff also cited the importance of consultation with pain care champions; access to on-site or nearby treatment services for pain care, such as pain management or other specialty clinics; or the role of clinical pharmacists. An additional asset to their work was the role of nurses or ancillary staff in coordinating pain care. When patients were asked which aspects of their pain care had gone particularly well, patients most frequently mentioned receiving effective treatment that relieved their pain and supported a return to previous activities. Patients also valued providers who listened to their concerns with a patient-centered approach. Some patients expressed confidence in their providers' ability to accurately diagnose and treat their pain, and some valued having access to multiple treatment options.

Staff and Patients Recommended Prioritizing Increases in Treatment Access and Availability to Improve Pain Care

When queried about barriers to delivering high-quality pain care, most staff cited appointment lengths that were too short to effectively manage patients with chronic pain, inadequate staffing to support service members' treatment needs, military-related issues, and the unavailability of some pain treatments and programs. Military-related issues included the stigma often associated with seeking pain care and the fear that time away from duties to receive that care could negatively affect a service member's career progression. Patients echoed many of these same barriers to care, including issues around access, such as long wait times for appointments; stigma associated with seeking pain care; challenges finding a provider and difficulty getting to appointments. When asked about recommendations to improve pain care delivered by the MHS, both staff and patients recommended increasing access to and availability of treatments. Staff recommended hiring more providers and increasing access to treatment, particularly for NPT. Patients also recommended improvements to increase access and availability of treatments and appointments. Providers recommended increasing provider training opportunities and cited the need for longer appointments, especially for adequate time to manage more-complex patient cases. Patients relatedly endorsed recommendations for providers' having enough time during an appointment to perform thorough examinations, offer counseling about treatment choices, and listen to patient concerns. Other top recommendations among staff included improving care coordination and continuity or increasing patient engagement in treatment, such as through education about what chronic pain is and which treatments might be appropriate. Some patients mentioned the need for improved care coordination or recommended a shift in military culture to decrease the perceived stigma associated with seeking pain care.

Recommendations

In this section, we provide recommendations to support the MHS in their efforts to continue to improve pain care delivered to service members. These recommendations are based on findings from our interviews and are also informed by findings and recommendations included in RAND's earlier report on quality of pain care delivered to service members (Hepner et al., 2022).

Recommendation 1. Increase Integration of Effective Nonpharmacologic Treatment

Recommendation 1a. Increase Access to Effective Nonpharmacologic Treatment

NPT is a strongly recommended first-line option for the treatment of chronic pain in multiple relevant VA/DoD CPGs (U.S. Department of Veterans Affairs and U.S. Department of Defense, 2020a; U.S. Department of Veterans Affairs and U.S. Department of Defense, 2022a; U.S. Department of Veterans Affairs and U.S. Department of Defense, 2022b), and its use is associated with fewer adverse outcomes in Army soldiers with chronic pain after transition to VA care (Meerwijk et al., 2020). Furthermore, the use of NPT is central to the MHS's implementation of the stepped-care model (Defense Health Agency Procedural Instruction 6025.04, 2018). Analyses of MHS administrative data indicated that the MHS should increase the delivery of NPT to support consistent implementation of the stepped-care model (Hepner et al., 2022). Increasing NPT access and appointment availability was among the most frequent recommendations made by staff and patients alike in our qualitative interviews. Most staff reported always integrating NPT into their treatment of patients with chronic pain, and most patients indicated that they preferred NPT. However, over three-quarters of staff described limited availability of NPT as the biggest barrier to integrating NPT into pain care. Other barriers that limited patients' access to NPT, as reported by staff, included inadequate staffing, long appointment wait times, and reimbursement issues related to private-sector care. Relatedly, more than half of patients stated that a lack of available appointments was a barrier to their pain care, although these comments were not exclusive to NPT. Phase 1 of this study found that some types of NPT were commonly delivered in the MHS—specifically, physical and occupational therapy, guided or supervised exercise, and chiropractic care and/or manipulation (Hepner et al., 2022). Other types of recommended NPT were less common, including acupuncture, biofeedback and/or hypnotherapy, and psychotherapy associated with a diagnosis of pain. In our interviews, providers were more likely to mention integrating BH care or psychotherapy for pain compared with the proportion of patients who reported receiving these NPTs as part of their treatment. Other types of recommended treatments, including cognitive behavioral therapy (a specific recommended type of psychotherapy for pain), tai chi, and yoga, were not coded in the administrative data, making it challenging to assess their utilization. However, only a limited number of providers and patients in our interviews indicated that these uncoded treatments were incorporated into their pain care. These findings highlight the need to increase access to NPT, particular on underutilized, recommended types of NPT.

There are several potential strategies that the MHS could pursue to increase access to NPT. Within MTFs, ensuring adequate staffing and appointment availability is critical. The MHS should assess whether there is adequate availability of the types of providers necessary to ensure timely access to NPT. In addition, a recent systematic review found that treatment models that included decision support that guided providers through a treatment algorithm or the stepped-care model, combined with proactive treatment monitoring, were most effective in improving pain and pain-related functioning (Peterson et al., 2017; Peterson et al., 2018). It may also be useful to leverage some of the more innovative practices highlighted by staff and patients, such as providing on-demand or "sick call" access to physical therapy for patients with chronic pain or increasing the use of embedded physical therapists, occupational therapists, or athletic trainers located in military units or in other places where services members may be more likely to be exposed to injuries that could result in chronic pain. Telehealth may also hold potential for increasing access to certain NPT (e.g., cognitive behavioral therapy for chronic pain), particularly for patients who face transportation barriers or are in regions with provider shortages (Byrne and Spevak, 2020; Mannes et al., 2022). Additionally, MTFs could provide protected training time and in-house training for providers, such as in battlefield acupuncture. In addition, research shows that the expansion of insurance coverage for NPT is associated with increased use (Choo et al., 2021; Mannes et al., 2022). Thus, it may be effective to expand TRICARE reimbursement to include such services as acupuncture and chiropractic care, which are not reimbursed if received through private-sector providers (TRICARE, 2020; TRICARE, 2022). Referrals to private-sector care for NPT could increase access when timely access is not available from an MTF provider. Finally, it could be useful for MTFs to establish a resource or designate an ancillary staff member with knowledge of local NPT resources.

Recommendation 1b. Monitor Access to Nonpharmacologic Treatment as Part of a Comprehensive Strategy to Improve the Quality of Pain Care

The monitoring of a system's quality of care can identify areas of high quality and those of lower quality to inform quality improvement efforts (Institute of Medicine et al., 2013). Ongoing monitoring of access and quality of care is essential to improving pain care delivered by the MHS. Both current and prior RAND findings highlight the need to increase access to NPT. Some types of NPT were integrated much more frequently (e.g., physical therapy), but several types of NPT were rarely integrated (e.g., acupuncture and psychotherapy associated with a pain diagnosis) (Hepner et al., 2022). The MHS monitors several metrics related to opioid prescribing using pharmacy data from both direct and private-sector care (U.S. Department of Defense, 2021). Perhaps because of this ongoing monitoring, the MHS performs quite well across most metrics related to appropriate opioid prescribing. The MHS should expand its monitoring and improvement efforts to include metrics that assess integration of NPT. Prior RAND work included several metrics that assessed quality of pain care, including the integration of NPT, and examined receipt of different type of recommended NPT (Hepner et al., 2022). Inclusion of one or more of these metrics may support monitoring of NPT delivery. Data about some aspects of pain care, such as treatments offered or referral to NPT, are not documented in coded administrative data, making monitoring more challenging. The use of the MHS GENESIS EHR and the continued implementation of clinical pathways to standardize pain management could also be used to collect and monitor data about pain treatments, including NPT.

Recommendation 2. Identify Barriers to Broader Use of the Defense and Veterans Pain Rating Scale

The DVPRS is the designated standard pain scale to be used by all providers (primary care and specialty) in MTFs to screen and assess for pain in adolescent and adult patients during each visit and guides the assessment of its impact on the service member's functioning (Defense Health Agency Procedural Instruction 6025.04, 2018). Although the MHS has rolled out the DVPRS to providers, our findings suggest that continued support is needed to increase its use. Specifically, only half of providers reported using a structured method to assess the impact of pain on patient functioning and response to treatment. The reasons for the lack of use of the DVPRS to assess the impact of pain on functioning are unclear, and further work is needed to understand the specific barriers impeding broader implementation of the DVPRS. It is possible that providers could benefit from additional education on the use of the DVPRS and its value. In addition, the DVPRS should be feasible to use and easily accessible in the medical record. The current transition to GENESIS provides an opportunity to continue to promote the use of structured and longitudinal evaluations of outcomes of treatment and to provide other pain treatment decision support. Increasing the use of a structured method, such as the DVPRS, to assess the impact of pain has several potential advantages. It allows the provider to implement measurement-based care—an approach in which structured measures are used to monitor changes in patient symptoms, inform treatment adjustment, and engage patients in their care. Furthermore, use of the DVPRS may increase the likelihood that the assessment of pain and the treatment provided are equitable among patients, regardless of patient background.

Recommendation 3. Expand Provider Education on Effective Treatment Options and Appropriate Opioid Prescribing

Interviews with both staff and patients highlighted the need for education on effective treatment for pain care. Increasing provider training and patient education in targeted areas is a strategy that may help support the MHS in its ongoing quality improvement efforts. Staff endorsed the value of access to provider training and consultative support for pain care. In the same vein, staff recommended increased access to provider training and improved provider awareness of pain treatment options. To support this need, the MHS should ensure that providers have protected time to attend training and that pain champions have time to support their providers. MHS could also leverage such existing programs as Project ECHO to provide training opportunities to staff. Staff from three different MTFs discussed the benefits of attending Project ECHO meetings, but it was not clear from our interviews whether such opportunities were available to providers at other MTFs. Providers and patients alike also cited the need for patient education on treatment options. Both provider education and patient education and activation are among the most common intervention components of multimodal chronic pain care (Peterson et al., 2017; Peterson et al., 2018). Thus, the MHS should increase provider training on the evidence base for types of NPT for different conditions. Providers may benefit from MTF-specific guidance on available types of NPT, how patients can be referred, and whom to contact when faced with access challenges. The MHS might also look for opportunities to involve nurses and medical technicians in the provision of patient education.

Furthermore, providers may need additional training on appropriate opioid prescribing—with an emphasis on how to prescribe for limited indications rather than solely on avoidance of prescribing. Administrators discussed the availability of provider training and the ability to consult with pain specialists and pain care champions as key supports for appropriate opioid prescribing. However, most interviewed providers indicated some level of uncertainty and discomfort with prescribing opioids and, therefore, may benefit from additional guidance on when it is appropriate to prescribe opioids to treat service members with acute or chronic pain and how to manage service members on LOT, including how to safely titrate patients off LOT, particularly given the risks of overdose and suicide risk with rapid titrations (U.S. Food & Drug Administration, 2019). Additionally, providers should receive education about treatment settings in which titration is and is not appropriate, particularly given recent evidence suggesting that there may be more harms (e.g., suicide and overdose) associated with opioid tapering compared with a stable opioid dosage (Larochelle et al., 2022). Pain care champions could be provided with additional training to serve as a resource for provider questions about LOT management and opioid titration and could facilitate the dissemination of additional guidance on opioid prescribing. This education could build on CPG content that offers talking points for providers when recommending changes to patients on opioids (U.S. Department of Veterans Affairs and U.S. Department of Defense, 2022b). Additionally, providers should be educated on when referrals to specialists should be made for complex opioid treatment cases based on a stepped-care model. In our earlier Phase 1 work, we found that receipt of recommended opioid prescribing for post-procedure pain was variable depending on the procedure performed. In addition, analyses revealed lower adherence to prescribing recommendations by private-sector providers compared with direct care providers (Hepner et al., 2022). Others have reported the variability of post-surgical procedure opioid prescribing among MHS dental clinics (Richard et al., 2021). We recommended providing more-precise and procedure-specific opioid prescribing guidelines to both MTF and private-sector providers.

Recommendation 4. Explore the Feasibility and Impact of Allowing Extended Visit Length for Primary Care Appointments for Patients with Complex Pain Needs

Staff members identified inadequate appointment length as the most common overarching barrier to delivering evidence-based pain care. Staff explained that the standard appointment length of 15 to 20 minutes was generally inadequate, particularly for patients with complex pain care needs. Providers discussed needing more time during the visit to obtain patient buy-in, provide education, and discuss treatment options. Patients similarly reported that inadequate appointment length was a common barrier, although this theme was more prominent as a recommendation: Patients discussed the need for longer appointments to allow time to have their concerns addressed as part of the development of a treatment plan. Nearly one-quarter of staff members recommended that appointments for chronic pain patients be longer. This finding is consistent with literature from civilian medicine that demonstrates that 20-minute appointment times are often too short to manage preventive care and chronic medical conditions (Yarnall et al., 2003). Patients have become more medically complex, treatment options more abundant, and the amount of data that clinicians need to absorb greater (Linzer et al., 2015). Inadequate time may lead to further clinician burnout, poorer quality of care, and reduced patient satisfaction (Linzer et al., 2009; Linzer et al., 2015; Howie et al., 1991). Our findings suggest that limiting primary care appointments to 20 minutes for patients with complex pain needs may limit providers' ability to educate and engage patients in their pain care and adequately address their complex needs. The MHS should explore the potential impact and feasibility of defining an enterprisewide appointment standard that allows for a small number of complex patient appointments in primary care that would be longer than the standard appointment length of 20 minutes. Additionally, the MHS may consider expanding patient visit time by involving nurses or case managers as part of the visit for patients with chronic pain. These providers could support the primary clinician in patient pain assessment, education, and referrals.

Recommendation 5. Improve Patient Experience in Receiving Care for Chronic Pain, and Ensure Pain Care Is Equitable

Patients identified several positive aspects of their care for chronic pain received from the MHS, including shared decisionmaking, being offered a choice of treatments, learning about risks and benefits of treatment options, and feeling that their provider listened to their preferences. But our interviews highlighted some areas in which patient experience could be improved. Specifically, patients report less favorable perceptions of coordination of care between their providers, and nearly one-quarter felt they had been treated differently because of some aspect of their background. These findings suggest that the MHS can continue to improve patient experience in receiving pain care and ensure that the care is delivered equitably.

Patients indicated that they valued care that involved communication about treatment options and shared decisionmaking in developing a treatment plan. Patients also voiced a desire for more awareness of treatment options, including NPT and techniques for pain self-management. Notably, providers indicated that patients did not always buy into or engage in recommended care. Providers may benefit from guidance and tools to engage patients in appropriate pain care and to communicate the effectiveness of NPT. Patients recommended increasing the use of diagnostic imaging, such as MRI—a perspective that is generally not consistent with recommendations in CPGs. Advanced imaging is recommended only with concerning physical exam findings (e.g., significant or progressive neurologic deficits), after treatment failures (e.g., lack of clinical improvement with NSAIDs or physical therapy), or in other unique situations (Chou et al., 2009; Jacobs et al., 2020; Jarvik et al., 2015; U.S. Department of Veterans Affairs and U.S. Department of Defense, 2022a). These patient perspectives may be due in part to a communication breakdown between patients and providers as to the appropriate use and timing of advanced imaging. Increasing provider training and available resources, such as patient education materials, would support providers in sharing evidence-based guidance on appropriate use of NPT and the role and timing of imaging in pain care. Nursing and ancillary staff could be utilized to provide patient education in clinical settings in addition to counseling from providers. Offering pain care education groups could provide another means of conveying information to patients about treatment options and best practices. Increased patient education and activation could support the initiation of pain care earlier, increase patient engagement in care, and improve patient experience.

It is important to ensure that care is delivered equitably, particularly given persistent disparities in pain care in the United States (Hoffman et al., 2016; Institute of Medicine, 2001; Meghani, Byun, and Gallagher, 2012). Yet nearly one-quarter of the patients with chronic pain who we interviewed believed that their pain care varied based on some aspect of their background. Using stratified reporting, quality metrics can be used to examine variations in pain care (Fiscella, Burstin, and Nerenz, 2014; Health Research & Educational Trust, 2014; Jha and Zaslavsky, 2014; Meghani et al., 2012; Simon et al., 2015). Should care vary by patient characteristics, these variations should be investigated for potential causes and quality improvement strategies implemented to minimize variation. For example, analyses of care for posttraumatic stress disorder and depression delivered to service members by the MHS revealed that some aspects of recommended care varied by service member characteristics (i.e., race and ethnicity, age, pay grade, deployment history), service branch, region, and whether a service member lived farther from an MTF (Hepner et al., 2021; Hepner et al., 2017; Hepner et al., 2016). Examination of quality metrics both for the MHS as a whole and stratified by key variables is an important tool to inform ongoing improvements in pain care.

Providers and patients both referred to tensions between receiving appropriate treatment for pain and fulfilling military duties. Patient experience could be improved by directly addressing these tensions, such as through improving access to on-demand NPT or making it easier to schedule appointments around military training and work schedules. Some aspects of military culture may be associated with stigma toward service members who seek treatment for pain. Service members may believe that acknowledging the impact of pain on functioning and seeking treatment reflects weakness, delaying care and exacerbating pain. Although provider education and patient resources may help address this issue, a meaningful shift in these perspectives will likely require a broader intervention across the military that includes both service members and their command.

Summary

Our interviews with MTF staff and service members receiving treatment at MTFs for chronic pain provided valuable context for the findings on pain care quality drawn from MHS administrative data in the first phase of this study. Administrative data capture patterns of care, offer insights into the extent to which service members receive evidence-based care, and are essential to measuring the quality of pain care in the MHS. Qualitative data provide a more complete picture of how the MHS organizes to provide pain care and how policies and guidance are implemented in practice and reveal facilitators and barriers to high-quality pain care at MTFs. The findings and recommendations in this report highlight areas for improvement and suggestions for innovation to ensure that the MHS continues providing timely, high-quality pain care that supports service members' outcomes and the readiness of the force.

Staff Interview Guide

Structured Items

Military service branch:
    a. Army
    b. Navy
    c. Marines
    d. Air Force

Status:
    a. Active component
    b. DoD government civilian
    c. Contractor (Note: Contactors are ineligible for the study. Please thank them for their time and do not interview.)

Rank (if applicable):
    a. O-1–O-2
    b. O-3–O-4
    c. O-5–O-6
    d. O-7–O-8

Do you currently have a clinical role, administrative role, or both?
    a. Clinical
    b. Administrative
    c. Both

Which types of outpatient clinics do you work in? *(Interviewer: Select all that apply.)*
    a. Primary care
    b. Pain management
    c. Physical medicine/rehabilitative care/occupational medicine/physical therapy
    d. Mental health specialty care
    e. Substance use disorder specialty care
    f. Integrated MH/substance use disorder care program

    g.   Pharmacy

    h.   Other: _____

What type of provider? *(Interviewer: Select the one that aligns most closely.)*

    a.   Primary care practitioner (MD, DO)

    b.   Pain medicine specialist

    c.   OB/GYN [obstetrics and gynecology] physician

    d.   Psychiatrist

    e.   Psychologist

    f.   LCSW [licensed clinical social worker]

    g.   Pharmacist

    h.   Physical therapist

    i.   Occupational therapist

    j.   Nurse (advanced practice or practitioner)

    k.   Physician assistant

    l.   Other: _____

Are you currently delivering or overseeing care for: *(Interviewer: Select all that apply.)*

    a.   Acute pain conditions

    b.   Chronic pain conditions

[For Provider Interviews Only] Which of the following treatments for pain are you currently providing to service members at this MTF? *(Interviewer: Select all that apply.)*

    a.   Opioid medication treatment

    b.   Non-opioid medication treatment

    c.   Non-pharmacologic therapies

    d.   Management of long-term opioid use (LOT generally refers to over 90 days of opioid therapy)

    e.   Medication treatment following procedures, such as surgical procedures

[For Provider Interviews Only] How many years have you been working as a military health provider?

    a.   _____ years

[For Provider Interviews Only] In your role as a military health provider, how often do you provide care for patients with acute or chronic pain conditions? On average . . .

    a.   Multiple patients per day

    b.   Multiple patients per week

    c.   Multiple patients per month

    d.   One patient per month or less frequently

Staff Interview: Semi-Structured Items

Probes associated with each question are example probes. Probes used by the interviewer will depend on the responses and unique experience of the respondent.

Overarching Approach to Pain Treatment

a. *[For providers]* Providing treatment for pain includes care for acute pain, lasting less than three months, and chronic pain, lasting three months or longer. Do you have a particular approach that guides your treatment of service members with pain? This could be an approach that you use or a program that has been adopted at this clinic or MTF. Please describe.

    i. *Probe:* Is this a structured approach or formal program?

    ii. *Probe:* Use one treatment at a time or multiple?

    iii. *[Optional] Probe:* Approach to adjusting or sequencing treatment?

b. *[For providers]* Does your approach vary based on whether the patient has acute pain or chronic pain?

c. *[For administrators]* Providing treatment for pain includes care for acute pain, lasting less than three months, and chronic pain, lasting three months or longer. Does this clinic or MTF have a particular approach that guides treatment of service members with pain? Please describe.

    i. *Probe:* Is this a structured approach or formal program?
       [Interviewer]: Document program features including model (e.g., stepped care, multimodal care, collaborative care), level/type of guidance, decision support, types of providers and clinics involved, associated training, etc.]

Treatment Selection and Shared Decision Making in Chronic Pain

a. *[For providers]* Next, let's focus on service members with chronic pain—pain lasting three months or longer. In treating a service member with chronic pain, what factors do you consider in developing a plan for treatment? This might include patient factors, treatment factors, policies, or how care is delivered at this clinic or MTF.

    i. *Probe (patient factors):* [e.g., factors related to patient presentation or patient preferences]
       Optional Examples: type and severity of condition, co-occurring mental health or substance use issues, patient preferences, past treatment received

    ii. *Probe (treatment factors):* [e.g., factors related to treatment options or guidelines]
       Optional Examples: effectiveness or safety of treatment options, MHS policy or clinical practice guideline

    iii. *Probe (organizational/structural factors):* [e.g., factors related to clinic operations or programs]

Optional Examples: availability of treatment options, formal program approach at MTF (stepped care approach, team-based care)

b. *[For providers]* In planning treatment for a service member with chronic pain, does the patient play a role in that process? Please describe.
   i. *[Optional] Probe:* Discuss options with patient, provide patient education, discuss risk/benefits, listen for patient concerns, preferences, or barriers?
   ii. *[Optional] Probe:* Any unique challenges in incorporating NPTs versus medications?

Non-Pharmacological Therapies
a. *[For providers]* Non-pharmacological therapies include a range of treatment such as exercise, physical therapy, occupational therapy, acupuncture, and psychotherapy. What influences whether you integrate non-pharmacological therapies to treat a service member with chronic pain?
   i. *Probe: Patient factors* [e.g., factors related to patient presentation or patient preferences]
   Optional Examples: (e.g., type of pain condition, patient characteristics or comorbidities, phase of treatment, patient perceptions or preferences)?
   ii. *Probe: Provider factors* [e.g., your own preferences and views of treatment]
   Optional Examples: (e.g., provider preferences, treatment effectiveness)?
   iii. *Probe: Structural/organizational factors* [e.g., factors related to clinic operations or programs]
   Optional Examples: (e.g., availability of appointments or clinical service)?
   iv. *Probe:* What factors increase the likelihood that you will recommend an NPT?

b. *[For providers]* How does this differ for service members with acute pain?
c. *[For providers]* Are there non-pharmacological therapies that you rely on most heavily? Why? Any you avoid? Why?
d. *[For administrators]* Non-pharmacological therapies include a range of treatment such as exercise, physical therapy, occupational therapy, acupuncture, and psychotherapy. To what degree do providers at this clinic or MTF integrate non-pharmacological therapies to treat a service member with chronic pain?
e. *[For providers/administrators]* What do you see as the biggest barrier in incorporating non-pharmacological therapies in the treatment of pain for service members?
f. *[For administrators]* Are there any processes in place to support providers in using non-pharmacological therapies for pain? This might include provider education, ongoing monitoring, or feedback.

Prescribing in Chronic Pain

a. *[For providers]* What influences whether you prescribe an opioid to treat a service member with chronic pain?

    i. *Probe: Patient factors* [e.g., factors related to patient presentation or patient preferences]
Optional Examples: (e.g., type of pain condition, patient characteristics or comorbidities, phase of treatment, patient perceptions or preferences)?

    ii. *Probe: Provider factors [e.g., your own preferences and views of treatment]*
Optional Examples: (e.g., provider preferences, treatment effectiveness)?

    iii. *Probe: Structural/organizational factors* [e.g., factors related to clinic operations or programs]
Optional Examples: (e.g., feedback about prescribing)?

b. *[For administrators]* Are there any processes in place to support providers to appropriately prescribe opioids for chronic pain? This might include provider education, ongoing monitoring, or feedback.

c. *[For providers]* Are there other prescription medications that you commonly use to treat chronic pain?

    i. *Probe:* Antidepressants? Gabapentin? Pregabalin?

    ii. *(If no) Probe:* Any particular reason why not?

Treatment Adjustment

a. *[For providers]* In treating a service member with chronic pain, what factors do you consider to inform whether current treatment needs to be adjusted, and what those adjustments should be?

    i. *[Optional] Probe:* Effectiveness of treatment, assessment of patient functioning/impact of pain, side effects, access/availability of treatment, patient preferences, stepped care

    ii. *Probe if not mentioned:* assessment of how pain affects the patient's daily activities?
[Interviewer: probe for detail on how pain assessment informs treatment adjustment, such as how assessed and how the information is used]

Barriers, Facilitators, and Recommendations

a. *[For providers/administrators]* What have you found helps or supports you (administrators: the providers you oversee) in being able to deliver high-quality care for acute and chronic pain?

    i. *Probes (structural/organizational supports):* [e.g., factors related to clinic operations or programs]

Optional Examples: team-based approach, provider-to-provider consultation with specialists, care coordination resources (e.g., nurse case managers), pharmacy-based feedback/oversight, EHR templates

   ii. *Probes (provider supports):* [e.g., factors related to your background, experience or preferences]
Optional Examples: training, experience with treatment options/NPTs

b. *[For providers/administrators]* What gets in the way of your ability (administrators: the ability of the providers you oversee) to deliver evidence-based treatment for acute and chronic pain? (Note any unique issues for different kinds of pain care.)

   i. *Probe (structural/organizational barriers):* [e.g., factors related to clinic operations or programs]
Optional Examples: Challenges in coordinating care, difficulty with EHR, availability of appointments?

   ii. *Probe (provider barriers):* [e.g., factors related to your background, experience or preferences]
Optional Examples: Training needs, preference for other treatments over NPTs?

   iii. *Probe (service member barriers):*
Optional Examples: Service member duties, time or financial barriers, perceptions about particular treatment options, stigma, unit/command issues)

c. *[For providers/administrators]* What recommendations do you have to overcome these barriers?

d. *[For providers/administrators]* Do you have any other comments on the topics we discussed today?

Patient Interview Guide

Structured Questions

Military service branch:
- a. Army
- b. Navy
- c. Marines
- d. Air Force

Status: *(Interviewer: Confirm that they are Active Component; all others are ineligible.)*
- a. Active component
- b. Other: _____

Rank (if applicable):
- a. E-1–E-4
- b. E-5–E-9
- c. O-1–O-3
- d. O-4–O-8

Race/ethnicity *(Interviewer: Select all that apply.)*
- a. American Indian or Alaska Native
- b. Asian
- c. Black or African American
- d. Hispanic or Latino origin or descent
- e. Native Hawaiian or Other Pacific Islander
- f. White
- g. None of these. Describe: _____

What is your military occupation? _____

Gender: _____

Age:

a. 18–24 years old
b. 25–34 years old
c. 35–44 years old
d. 45–54 years old
e. 55–64 years old

Which pain conditions have you been diagnosed with? *(Interviewer: Select all that apply.)*
a. Low Back Pain
b. Neck Pain
c. Fibromyalgia
d. Other musculoskeletal pain (bone, muscle, or joint pain): Specify: _____

In which types of settings have you received care for pain? *(Interviewer: Select all that apply.)*
a. Primary care
b. Occupational therapy/Physical therapy/Physical medicine/Rehabilitative care
c. Specialty pain care clinic
d. Behavioral health
e. Other—please specify: _____

How long have you been receiving treatment for this/these pain condition(s)? _____ (in months)

How long have you been receiving treatment for this/these pain condition(s) at this MTF? _____ (in months)

Patient Interview: Semi-Structured Items
Probes associated with each question are example probes. Probes used by the interviewer will depend on the responses and unique experience of the respondent.

a. I'd like to learn about the types of treatments have you received for pain. Focusing on the past six months, what types of treatments for pain have you received?
  i. *Probe:* Medications (non-opioids, opioids), non-pharmacological therapies?

Treatment Selection and Shared Decision Making

a. Do you recall talking with any provider about different treatments that could be used to treat your pain? What do you recall about these discussions?
  i. *Probe:* Offered choice of treatments?
  ii. *Probe:* Explained benefits and risks of each treatment?

    iii.   *Probe:* Recommend one type of treatment over another (i.e., medications vs. NPT)?

    iv.   *Probe:* Listened to patient's preferences?

Patient Perceptions of Treatment Options

a.   Treatment for pain can include a variety of treatments including medication and non-medication treatments like physical therapy, acupuncture, and cognitive behavioral therapy. As you considered possible treatments with your provider(s), did you have preferences or thoughts about different treatment options?

    i.   *Probe:* Preference for medication versus NPT?

    ii.   *Probe:* Preference for particular treatments? What treatment and why?

    iii.   *Probe:* Concerns about particular treatments (e.g., side effects, time or cost involved, stigma)?

    iv.   *Probe:* Treatment that provider recommended but patient declined? Why?

Barriers to Care (Access, Patient Barriers)

a.   [Focusing on the past six months] What has your experience been in receiving treatment for pain at this MTF? Has anything gotten in the way? [*Interviewer: Assess whether barriers are unique to NPT or particular NPTs.*]

    i.   *Probe:* Finding a provider or where to get care?

    ii.   *Probe:* Available appointments, wait times?

    iii.   *Probe:* Getting to appointments (getting away from duties, travel time)?

    iv.   *Probe:* Cost?

    v.   *Probe:* Stigma?

Coordination of Care

a.   Has there been a time in your pain care at this MTF when you had more than one provider treating your pain [at the same time]? If so, do you feel like they communicated well with each other about your care? (Interviewer: Assess for differences in communication within a clinic vs. communication with specialists.)

    i.   *Probe:* What indicated that there was communication?

    ii.   *Probe:* Adequacy of communication

Pain Assessment and Treatment Adjustment

a.   Did any provider who treats your pain ask about how pain affects you and your daily activities?

    i.   *Probe:* Frequency of pain assessment?

    ii.   *Probe:* One provider or multiple providers?

  b. For some patients, pain treatment can involve making changes to treatment or trying different treatments. Examples of these changes are a change in the dose of medication, the type of medication, or trying a non-medication treatment like physical therapy. [Focusing on the past six months] Did any of your providers make changes like this during your pain care? If so, please describe.

  c. What do you think was the reason for these changes?
    i.   *Probe:* treatment not effective, side effects, patient not adherent to treatment, trying a different "stronger" treatment

  d. Do you think your provider used their understanding of the impact of pain on your daily activities to change your treatment?

Equity

  a. This MTF provides pain care for service members from many different backgrounds. For example, service members are different in their age, race, ethnicity, gender, rank, sexual identity and orientation, religion, and income. Do you feel that you have been treated differently, or the types of pain care you have been offered have been different, because of your background?
    i.   *Probe:* In what ways?

Strengths and Areas for Improvement in Pain Care at this MTF

  a. Overall [focusing on the past six months], what aspects of your pain care do you feel have gone particularly well at this MTF?
  b. How do you think pain care could be improved at this MTF?
  c. Do you have any other comments on the topics we discussed today?

Selected Reviews of Effectiveness of Models of Care

Table C.1 provides an overview of our systematic review.

TABLE C.1

Selected Systematic Reviews of Effectiveness of Models to Deliver Multimodal Pain Care

Author and Year	Model	Patient Population	Studies	End Date of Review	Care Settings	Study Countries	Measured Outcomes	Findings
Elbers et al., 2022	Interdisciplinary, multimodal: biopsychosocial model of pain, active patient participation, at least three different health care professionals, single facility of care	Chronic primary musculoskeletal pain	37 case series, 20 RCTs, 4 N-RCTs, 5 other study design	May 2020	Most in secondary or tertiary care	Europe, Australia, Canada	At least one of the following: physical functioning, pain interference, depression, anxiety, emotional functioning, anger, self-efficacy, social functioning, pain intensity	Majority of patient cohorts significantly improved between pre- to posttreatment.
Peterson et al., 2017; Peterson et al., 2018	Any model with system-based mechanisms to increase uptake and organization of multimodal care	Chronic primary musculoskeletal pain	8 RCTs, 1 retrospective cohort study	October 2016	Integrated within primary care	Mostly United States, including four VA Medical Centers; Canada; United Kingdom	Reduction in pain intensity and pain-related function from baseline of at least 30 percent or 50 percent, quality of life, depression, anxiety, sleep, opioid doses	Five models with decision support coupled with proactive treatment monitoring had the strongest evidence of clinically important improvements in pain and function.
Saracoglu, Akin, and Aydin Dincer, 2022	Multimodal with added pain neuroscience education	Fibromyalgia	4 RCTs	June 2021	Primary care and/ or physical therapy	Spain	Severity of fibromyalgia, pain intensity, catastrophizing, depression, anxiety	Groups with pain neuroscience education were statistically more effective in improving outcomes.
Sutton et al., 2016	Multimodal: two distinct therapeutic modalities provided by one or more disciplines	Whiplash-associated disorders or neck pain	14 RCTs	May 2013	Most in physical therapy	Europe, Australia	Self-rated recovery, function, pain intensity, health-related quality of life, psychological outcomes	Evidence did not indicate that one multimodal package was superior to another.

NOTE: RCT = randomized controlled trials.

Abbreviations

AHLTA	Armed Forces Health Longitudinal Technology Application
BH	behavioral health
CME	continuing medical education
COVID-19	coronavirus disease 2019
CPG	clinical practice guideline
DHA	Defense Health Agency
DO	doctor of osteopathic medicine
DoD	U.S. Department of Defense
DVPRS	Defense and Veterans Pain Rating Scale
ECHO	Extension for Community Healthcare Outcomes
EHR	electronic health record
ER	emergency room
FY	fiscal year
IBHC	integrated behavioral health consultant
IPMC	interdisciplinary pain management center
LOT	long-term opioid therapy
MD	doctor of medicine
MEDD	morphine equivalent daily dose
MHS	Military Health System
MME	morphine milligram equivalent
MOS	military occupational specialty
MOTION	Military Orthopedics Tracking Injuries and Outcomes Network
MRI	magnetic resonance imaging
MTF	military treatment facility
NPT	nonpharmacologic treatment
NSAID	nonsteroidal anti-inflammatory drug
OUD	opioid use disorder
PASTOR	Pain Assessment Screening Tool and Outcomes Registry
PCM	primary care manager
PCMH	patient-centered medical home
SD	standard deviation
SOCOM	Special Operations Command
TENS	transcutaneous electrical nerve stimulation
VA	U.S. Department of Veterans Affairs

References

American Dental Association, "Acute Dental Pain Management Guideline (2023)," webpage, 2023. As of March 2, 2023
https://www.ada.org/resources/research/science-and-research-institute/
evidence-based-dental-research/pain-management-guideline

Army Regulation 600-85, *The Army Substance Abuse Program*, Headquarters Department of the Army, July 23, 2020.

Bader, Christine E., Nicholas A. Giordano, Catherine C. McDonald, Salimah H. Meghani, and Rosemary C. Polomano, "Musculoskeletal Pain and Headache in the Active Duty Military Population: An Integrative Review," *Worldviews on Evidence-Based Nursing*, Vol. 15, No. 4, 2018.

Blakey, Shannon M., H. Ryan Wagner, Jennifer Naylor, Mira Brancu, Ilana Lane, Meghann Sallee, Nathan A. Kimbrel, Department of Veterans Affairs Mid-Atlantic Mental Illness Research, Education and Clinical Center Workgroup, and Eric B. Elbogen, "Chronic Pain, TBI, and PTSD in Military Veterans: A Link to Suicidal Ideation and Violent Impulses?" *Journal of Pain*, Vol. 19, No. 7, 2018.

Bradley, Elizabeth H., Leslie A. Curry, Shoba Ramanadhan, Laura Rowe, Ingrid M. Nembhard, and Harlan M. Krumholz, "Research in Action: Using Positive Deviance to Improve Quality of Health Care," *Implementation Science*, Vol. 4, May 2009.

Briggs, Andrew M., Peter Bragge, Helen Slater, Madelynn Chan, and Simon C. B. Towler, "Applying a Health Network Approach to Translate Evidence-Informed Policy into Practice: A Review and Case Study on Musculoskeletal Health," *BMC Health Services Research*, Vol. 12, November 2012.

Briggs, Andrew M., Madelynn Chan, and Helen Slater, "Models of Care for Musculoskeletal Health: Moving Towards Meaningful Implementation and Evaluation Across Conditions and Care Settings," *Best Practice & Research Clinical Rheumatology*, Vol. 30, No. 3, 2016.

Buckenmaier, Chester, *Army Pain Management Task Force: Findings-Recommendations-Way Ahead*, U.S. Department of the Army, 2010.

Byrne, Taylor, and Christopher Spevak, "The Use of Telepain for Chronic Pain in the U.S. Armed Forces: Patient Experience from Walter Reed National Military Medical Center," *Military Medicine*, Vol. 185, No. 5/6, 2020.

Choo, Esther K., Christina J. Charlesworth, Yifan Gu, Catherine J. Livingston, and K. John McConnell, "Increased Use of Complementary and Alternative Therapies for Back Pain Following Statewide Medicaid Coverage Changes in Oregon," *Journal of General Internal Medicine*, Vol. 36, March 2021.

Chou, Roger, Rongwei Fu, John A. Carrino, and Richard A. Deyo, "Imaging Strategies for Low-Back Pain: Systematic Review and Meta-Analysis," *Lancet*, Vol. 373, February 2009.

Chun Tie, Ylona, Melanie Birks, and Karen Francis, "Grounded Theory Research: A Design Framework for Novice Researchers," *SAGE Open Medicine*, Vol. 7, January 2019.

Cordts, Paul R., and Defense Health Agency, "Integration of the Pain Assessment Screening Tool and Outcomes Registry (PASTOR) into Daily Clinical Practice," memorandum to DHA Markets and Military Medical Treatment Facilities (MTFS), May 11, 2022.

Defense Health Agency, "Fact Sheet: PASTOR," March 2018. As of January 17, 2023:
https://www.health.mil/Reference-Center/Fact-Sheets/2018/03/26/PASTOR-Fact-Sheet

Defense Health Agency Procedural Instruction 6010.02, *Military Health System Prescription Drug Monitoring Program*, Department of Defense, October 15, 2021.

Defense Health Agency Procedural Instruction 6025.04, *Pain Management and Opioid Safety in the Military Health System (MHS)*, June 18, 2018.

Defense Health Agency Procedural Instruction 6025.27, *Integration of Primary Care Behavioral Health (PCBH) Services into Patient-Centered Medical Home (PCMH) and Other Primary Care Service Settings Within the Military Health System (MHS)*, Department of Defense, 2019.

Defense Health Agency Procedural Instruction 6025.33, *Acupuncture Practice in Military Medical Treatment Facilities (MTFs)*, Department of Defense, 2020.

Department of the Army Pamphlet 611-21, *Personnel Selection and Classification: Military Occupational Classification and Structure*, Headquarters Department of the Army, July 19, 2018.

Dowell, Deborah, Kathleen R. Ragan, Christopher M. Jones, Grant T. Baldwin, and Roger Chou, "CDC Clinical Practice Guideline for Prescribing Opioids for Pain—United States, 2022," Morbidity and Mortality Weekly Report, Vol. 71, No. 3, November 4, 2022.

Elbers, Stefan, Harriët Wittink, Sophie Konings, Ulrike Kaiser, Jos Kleijnen, Jan Pool, Albère Köke, and Rob Smeets, "Longitudinal Outcome Evaluations of Interdisciplinary Multimodal Pain Treatment Programmes for Patients with Chronic Primary Musculoskeletal Pain: A Systematic Review and Meta-Analysis," *European Journal of Pain*, Vol. 26, No. 2, 2022.

Farooqi, Owais A., W. E. Bruhn, M. K. Lecholop, D. Velasquez-Plata, J. G. Maloney, S. Rizwi, R. B. Templeton, A. Goerig, C. Hezkial, C. M. Novince, M. T. Zieman, A. M. N. Lotesto, and M. A. Makary, "Opioid Guidelines for Common Dental Surgical Procedures: A Multidisciplinary Panel Consensus," *International Journal of Oral Maxillofacial Surgery*, Vol. 49, No. 3, 2020.

Fiscella, Kevin, Helen R. Burstin, and David R. Nerenz, "Quality Measures and Sociodemographic Risk Factors: To Adjust or Not to Adjust," *JAMA*, Vol. 312, No. 24, 2014.

Flynn, Diane M., Karon Cook, Michael Kallen, Chester Buckenmaier, Ricke Weickum, Teresa Collins, Ashley Johnson, Dawn Morgan, Kevin Galloway, and Kristin Joltes, "Use of the Pain Assessment Screening Tool and Outcomes Registry in an Army Interdisciplinary Pain Management Center, Lessons Learned and Future Implications of a 10-Month Beta Test," *Military Medicine*, Vol. 182, No. S1, 2017.

Garvin, Jennifer, "ADA Adopts Interim Opioids Policy," *ADA News*, March 29, 2018.

Guise, Jeanne-Marie, Christine Chang, Meera Viswanathan, Susan Glick, Jonathan Treadwell, Craig A. Umscheid, Evelyn Whitlock, Rochelle Fu, Elise Berliner, Robin Paynter, Johanna Anderson, Pua Motu'apuaka, and Tom Trikalinos, *Systematic Reviews of Complex Multicomponent Health Care Interventions*, Agency for Healthcare Research and Quality, March 2014.

Haibach, Jeffrey P., Gregory P. Beehler, Katherine M. Dollar, and Deborah S. Finnell, "Moving Toward Integrated Behavioral Intervention for Treating Multimorbidity Among Chronic Pain, Depression, and Substance-Use Disorders in Primary Care," *Medical Care*, Vol. 52, No. 4, 2014.

Health Research & Educational Trust, *A Framework for Stratifying Race, Ethnicity and Language Data*, October 2014.

Hepner, Kimberly A., Ryan Andrew Brown, Carol P. Roth, Teague Ruder, and Harold Alan Pincus, *Behavioral Health Care in the Military Health System: Access and Quality for Remote Service Members*, RAND Corporation, RR-2788-OSD, 2021. As of January 17, 2023: https://www.rand.org/pubs/research_reports/RR2788.html

Hepner, Kimberly A., Carol P. Roth, Tisamarie B. Sherry, Ryan K. McBain, Teague Ruder, and Charles C. Engel, *Assessing the Quality of Outpatient Pain Care and Opioid Prescribing in the Military Health System*, RAND Corporation, RR-A1193-1, 2022. As of January 17, 2023: https://www.rand.org/pubs/research_reports/RRA1193-1.html

Hepner, Kimberly A., Carol P. Roth, Elizabeth M. Sloss, Susan M. Paddock, Praise O. Iyiewuare, Martha J. Timmer, and Harold Alan Pincus, *Quality of Care for PTSD and Depression in the Military Health System: Final Report*, RAND Corporation, RR-1542-OSD, 2017. As of January 27, 2021: https://www.rand.org/pubs/research_reports/RR1542.html

Hepner, Kimberly A., Carol P. Roth, Jessica L. Sousa, Teague Ruder, Ryan Andrew Brown, Layla Parast, and Harold Alan Pincus, *Behavioral Health Care Delivery Following the Onset of the COVID-19 Pandemic: Utilization, Telehealth, and Quality of Care for Service Members with PTSD, Depression, or Substance Use Disorder*, RAND Corporation, RR-A412=3, 2023. As of June 22, 2023: https://www.rand.org/pubs/research_reports/RRA421-3.html

Hepner, Kimberly A., Elizabeth M. Sloss, Carol P. Roth, Heather Krull, Susan M. Paddock, Shaela Moen, Martha J. Timmer, and Harold Alan Pincus, *Quality of Care for PTSD and Depression in the Military Health System: Phase I Report*, RAND Corporation, RR-978-OSD, 2016. As of January 17, 2023: https://www.rand.org/pubs/research_reports/RR978.html

Hoffman, Kelly M., Sophie Trawalter, Jordan R. Axt, and M. Norman Oliver, "Racial Bias in Pain Assessment and Treatment Recommendations, and False Beliefs About Biological Differences Between Blacks and Whites," *Proceedings of the National Academy of Sciences*, Vol. 113, No. 16, 2016.

Howie, J. G. R., A. M. D. Porter, D. J. Heaney, and J. L. Hopton, "Long to Short Consultation Ratio: A Proxy Measure of Quality of Care for General Practice," *British Journal of General Practice*, Vol. 41, No. 343, 1991.

Human Performance Resources, "Physical Fitness: Rx3," webpage, Consortium for Health and Military Performance, undated. As of January 17, 2023: https://www.hprc-online.org/physical-fitness/rx3

Institute of Medicine, *Crossing the Quality Chasm: A New Health System for the 21st Century*, National Academies Press, 2001.

Institute of Medicine, *Relieving Pain in America: A Blueprint for Transforming Prevention, Care, Education, and Research*, National Academies Press, 2011.

Institute of Medicine, Mark Smith, Robert Saunders, Leigh Stuckhardt, and J. Michael McGinnis, eds., *Best Care at Lower Cost: The Path to Continuously Learning Health Care in America*, National Academies Press, 2013.

Jacobs, Josephine C., Jeffrey G. Jarvik, Roger Chou, Derek Boothroyd, Jeanie Lo, Andrea Nevedal, and Paul G. Barnett, "Observational Study of the Downstream Consequences of Inappropriate MRI of the Lumbar Spine," *Journal of General Internal Medicine*, Vol. 35, No. 12, 2020.

Jarvik, Jeffrey G., Laura S. Gold, Bryan A. Comstock, Patrick J. Heagerty, Sean D. Rundell, Judith A. Turner, Andrew L. Avins, Zoya Bauer, Brian W. Bresnahan, Janna L. Friedly, Kathryn James, Larry Kessler, Srdjan S. Nedeljkovic, David R. Nerenz, Xu Shi, Sean D. Sullivan, Leighton Chan, Jason M. Schwalb, and Richard A. Deyo, "Association of Early Imaging for Back Pain With Clinical Outcomes in Older Adults," *JAMA*, Vol. 313, No. 11, 2015.

Jha, Ashish K., and Alan M. Zaslavsky, "Quality Reporting That Addresses Disparities in Health Care," *JAMA*, Vol. 312, No. 3, 2014.

Kottke, Thomas E., Milo L. Brekke, and Leif I. Solberg, "Making 'Time' for Preventive Services," *Mayo Clinic Proceedings*, Vol. 68, No. 8, 1993.

Kwon, Edward, Christopher Stange, Katy Reichlin, Hamilton Vernon, Akira Miyanari, Elizabeth Bier, Hind Beydoun, and Virginia Kalish, "A Comprehensive, Multimodal, Interdisciplinary Approach to Chronic Non-Cancer Pain Management in a Family Medicine Clinic: A Retrospective Cohort Review," *Permanente Journal*, Vol. 25, No. 4, 2021.

Larochelle, Marc R., Sara Lodi, Shapei Yan, Barbara A. Clothier, Elizabeth S. Goldsmith, and Amy S. B. Bohnert, "Comparative Effectiveness of Opioid Tapering or Abrupt Discontinuation vs No Dosage Change for Opioid Overdose or Suicide for Patients Receiving Stable Long-Term Opioid Therapy," *JAMA Network Open*, Vol. 5, No. 8, 2022.

Lew, Henry L., John D. Otis, Carlos Tun, Robert D. Kerns, Michael E. Clark, and David X. Cifu, "Prevalence of Chronic Pain, Posttraumatic Stress Disorder, and Persistent Postconcussive Symptoms in OIF/OEF Veterans: Polytrauma Clinical Triad," *Journal of Rehabilitation Research Development*, Vol. 46, No. 6, 2009.

Linzer, Mark, Linda Baier Manwell, Eric S. Williams, James A. Bobula, Roger L. Brown, Anita B. Varkey, Bernice Man, Julia E. McMurray, Ann Maguire, Barbara Horner-Ibler, Mark D. Schwartz, and Minimizing Error, Maximizing Outcome Investigators, "Working Conditions in Primary Care: Physician Reactions and Care Quality," *Annals of Internal Medicine*, Vol. 151, No. 1, 2009.

Linzer, Mark, Asaf Bitton, Shin-Ping Tu, Margaret Plews-Ogan, Karen R. Horowitz, Mark D. Schwartz, and Association of Chiefs and Group Leaders in General Internal Medicine Writing Group, "The End of the 15–20 Minute Primary Care Visit," *Journal of General Internal Medicine*, Vol. 30, No. 11, 2015.

Mannes, Zachary L., Malki Stohl, David S. Fink, Mark Olfson, Katherine M. Keyes, Silvia S. Martins, Jaimie L. Gradus, Andrew J. Saxon, Charles Maynard, Ofir Livne, Sarah Gutkind, and Deborah S. Hasin, "Non-Pharmacological Treatment for Chronic Pain in US Veterans Treated Within the Veterans Health Administration: Implications for Expansion in US Healthcare Systems," *Journal of General Internal Medicine*, Vol. 37, No. 15, 2022.

Meerwijk, Esther L., Mary Jo Larson, Eric M. Schmidt, Rachel Sayko Adams, Mark R. Bauer, Grant A. Ritter, Chester Buckenmaier III, and Alex H. S. Harris, "Nonpharmacological Treatment of Army Service Members with Chronic Pain Is Associated with Fewer Adverse Outcomes After Transition to the Veterans Health Administration," *Journal of General Internal Medicine*, Vol. 35, No. 3, 2020.

Meghani, Salimah H., Eeeseung Byun, and Rollin M. Gallagher, "Time to Take Stock: A Meta-Analysis and Systematic Review of Analgesic Treatment Disparities for Pain in the United States," *Pain Medicine*, Vol. 13, No. 2, 2012.

Meghani, Salimah H., Rosemary C. Polomano, Raymond C. Tait, April H. Vallerand, Karen O. Anderson, and Rollin M. Gallagher, "Advancing a National Agenda to Eliminate Disparities in Pain Care: Directions for Health Policy, Education, Practice, and Research," *Pain Medicine*, Vol. 13, No. 1, 2012.

Military Health System, "MHS GENESIS: The Electronic Health Record," 2022. As of March 2, 2023:
https://www.health.mil/Military-Health-Topics/Technology/MHS-GENESIS

Neprash, Hannah T., Alexander Everhart, Donna McAlpine, Laura Barrie Smith, Bethany Sheridan, and Dori A. Cross, "Measuring Primary Care Exam Length Using Electronic Health Record Data," *Medical Care*, Vol. 59, No. 1, 2021.

Norcini, John J. Jr., "Standards and Reliability in Evaluation: When Rules of Thumb Don't Apply," *Academic Medicine*, Vol. 74, No. 10, 1999.

Overton, Heidi N., Marie N. Hanna, William E. Bruhn, Susan Hutfless, Mark C. Bicket, and Martin A. Makary, "Opioid-Prescribing Guidelines for Common Surgical Procedures: An Expert Panel Consensus," *Journal of the American College of Surgeons*, Vol. 227, No. 4, 2018.

Pakieser, Jennifer, Sidney Peters, Laura C. Tilley, Ryan C. Costantino, Maya Scott-Richardson, and Krista B. Highland, "Naloxone Prescribing Practices in the Military Health System Before and After Policy Implementation," *PAIN Reports*, Vol. 7, No. 2, 2021.

Peterson, Kim, Johanna Anderson, Donald Bourne, Katherine Mackey, and Mark Helfand, *Evidence Brief: Effectiveness of Models Used to Deliver Multimodal Care for Chronic Musculoskeletal Pain*, U.S. Department of Veterans Affairs, January 2017.

Peterson, Kim, Johanna Anderson, Donald Bourne, Katherine Mackey, and Mark Helfand, "Effectiveness of Models Used to Deliver Multimodal Care for Chronic Musculoskeletal Pain: A Rapid Evidence Review," *Journal of General Internal Medicine*, Vol. 33, Supplement 1, 2018.

Reif, Sharon, Rachel Sayko Adams, Grant A. Ritter, Thomas V. Williams, and Mary Jo Larson, "Prevalence of Pain Diagnoses and Burden of Pain Among Active Duty Soldiers, FY2012," *Military Medicine*, Vol. 183, No. 9/10, 2018.

Richard, Patrick, Mark R. Bauer, Natalie Moresco, Regine Walker, Diana Bowser, Demarcio Reed, and Mary Jo Larson, "Opioid Prescribing for Surgical Dental Procedures in Dental Clinics of Military Treatment Facilities," *Journal of the American Dental Association*, Vol. 152, No. 2, 2021.

Rose, Adam J., and Megan B. McCullough, "A Practical Guide to Using the Positive Deviance Method in Health Services Research," *Health Services Research*, Vol. 52, No. 3, 2017.

Saracoglu, Ismail, Esra Akin, and Gökce Basak Aydin Dincer, "Efficacy of Adding Pain Neuroscience Education to a Multimodal Treatment in Fibromyalgia: A Systematic Review and Meta-Analysis," *International Journal of Rheumatic Diseases*, Vol. 25, No. 4, 2022.

Sherry, Tisamarie B., Carol P. Roth, Mallika Bhandarkar, and Kimberly A. Hepner, *Chronic Pain Among Service Members: Using Administrative Data to Strengthen Research and Quality Improvement*, RAND Corporation, RR-A1160-1, 2021. As of January 17, 2023: https://www.rand.org/pubs/research_reports/RRA1160-1.html

Simon, Gregory E., Karen J. Coleman, Beth E. Waitzfelder, Arne Beck, Rebecca C. Rossom, Christine Stewart, and Robert B. Penfold, "Adjusting Antidepressant Quality Measures for Race and Ethnicity," *JAMA Psychiatry*, Vol. 72, No. 10, 2015.

Sokol, Randi G., Rachyl Pines, and Aaronson Chew, "Multidisciplinary Approach for Managing Complex Pain and Addiction in Primary Care: A Qualitative Study," *Annals of Family Medicine*, Vol. 19, No. 3, 2021.

Speerin, Robyn, Helen Slater, Linda Li, Karina Moore, Madelynn Chan, Karsten Dreinhöfer, Peter R. Ebeling, Simon Willcock, and Andrew M. Briggs, "Moving from Evidence to Practice: Models of Care for the Prevention and Management of Musculoskeletal Conditions," *Best Practice & Research: Clinical Rheumatology*, Vol. 28, No. 3, 2014.

Suman, Arnela, Marije F. Dikkers, Frederieke G. Schaafsma, Maurits W. van Tulder, and Johannes R. Anema, "Effectiveness of Multifaceted Implementation Strategies for the Implementation of Back and Neck Pain Guidelines in Health Care: A Systematic Review," *Implementation Science*, Vol. 11, No. 1, 2016.

Sutton, Deborah A., Pierre Côté, Jessica J. Wong, Sharanya Varatharajan, Kristi A. Randhawa, Hainan Yu, Danielle Southerst, Heather M. Shearer, Gabrielle M. van der Velde, Margareta C. Nordin, Linda J. Carroll, Silvano A. Mior, Anne L. Taylor-Vaisey, and Maja Stupar, "Is Multimodal Care Effective for the Management of Patients with Whiplash-Associated Disorders or Neck Pain and Associated Disorders? A Systematic Review by the Ontario Protocol for Traffic Injury Management (OPTIMa) Collaboration," *Spine Journal*, Vol. 16, No. 12, 2016.

Thomas, James, and Angela Harden, "Methods for the Thematic Synthesis of Qualitative Research in Systematic Reviews," *BMC Medical Research Methodology*, Vol. 8, July 2008.

TRICARE, "Covered Services: Acupuncture," updated June 18, 2020. As of January 17, 2023:
https://www.tricare.mil/CoveredServices/IsItCovered/Acupuncture

TRICARE, "Covered Services: Chiropractic Care," updated March 20, 2022. As of January 17, 2023:
https://www.tricare.mil/CoveredServices/IsItCovered/ChiropracticCare

U.S. Army Public Health Center, *2020 Health of the Force: Create a Healthier Force for Tomorrow*, 2020.

U.S. Department of Defense, *Report to Committees on Armed Services of the Senate and the House of Representatives: The Implementation of a Comprehensive Policy on Pain Management by the Military Health Care System for Fiscal Year 2021*, Office of the Secretary of Defense, June 17, 2021.

U.S. Department of Defense and U.S. Department of Veterans Affairs, "Defense and Veterans Pain Rating Scale," undated.
https://www.va.gov/PAINMANAGEMENT/docs/DVPRS_2slides_and_references.pdf

U.S. Department of Defense and U.S. Department of Veterans Affairs, *Pain Management Task Force: Final Report. Providing a Standardized DoD and VHA Vision and Approach to Pain Management to Optimize the Care for Warriors and Their Families*, Office of the Army Surgeon General, May 2010.

U.S. Department of Defense Instruction 6490.15, *Integration of Behavioral Health Personnel (BHP) Services into Patient-Centered Medical Home (PCMH) Primary Care and Other Primary Care Service Settings*, August 8, 2013.
https://www.esd.whs.mil/Portals/54/Documents/DD/issuances/dodi/649015p.pdf

U.S. Department of Veterans Affairs and U.S. Department of Defense, "VA/DoD Clinical Practice Guidelines," webpage, undated. As of January 19, 2023:
https://www.healthquality.va.gov/

U.S. Department of Veterans Affairs and U.S. Department of Defense, *VA/DoD Clinical Practice Guideline for the Non-Surgical Management of Hip & Knee Osteoarthritis*, Version 1.0, 2014.

U.S. Department of Veterans Affairs and U.S. Department of Defense, *VA/DoD Clinical Practice Guideline for Diagnosis and Treatment of Low Back Pain*, Version 2.0, September, 2017a.

U.S. Department of Veterans Affairs and U.S. Department of Defense, *VA/DoD Clinical Practice Guideline for Opioid Therapy for Chronic Pain*, Version 3.0, February, 2017b.

U.S. Department of Veterans Affairs and U.S. Department of Defense, *VA/DoD Clinical Practice Guideline for the Non-Surgical Management of Hip & Knee Osteoarthritis*, Version 2.0, July 2020a.

U.S. Department of Veterans Affairs and U.S. Department of Defense, *VA/DoD Clinical Practice Guideline for the Primary Care Management of Headache*, Version 1.0, July 2020b.

U.S. Department of Veterans Affairs and U.S. Department of Defense, *VA/DoD Clinical Practice Guideline for the Diagnosis and Treatment of Low Back Pain*, Version 3.0, February 2022a.

U.S. Department of Veterans Affairs and U.S. Department of Defense, *VA/DoD Clinical Practice Guideline for Use of Opioids in the Management of Chronic Pain*, Version 4.0, May 2022b.

U.S. Food & Drug Administration, "FDA Identifies Harm Reported from Sudden Discontinuation of Opioid Pain Medicines and Requires Label Changes to Guide Prescribers on Gradual, Individualized Tapering," April 9, 2019.

Von Korff, Michael, and Bea Tiemens, "Individualized Stepped Care of Chronic Illness," *Western Journal of Medicine*, Vol. 172, No. 2, 2000.

Yarnall, Kimberly S. H., Kathryn I. Pollak, Truls Østbye, Katrina M. Krause, and J. Lloyd Michener, "Primary Care: Is There Enough Time for Prevention?" *American Journal of Public Health*, Vol. 93, No. 4, 2003.